HISPANICS AND MENTAL HEALTH:
A Framework for Research

HISPANICS AND MENTAL HEALTH:
A Framework for Research

Lloyd H. Rogler

Albert Schweitzer University Professor
Director, Hispanic Research Center
Fordham University

Robert G. Malgady

Professor, Department of Mathematics, Science and Statistics
New York University
Research Associate, Hispanic Research Center
Fordham University

Orlando Rodriguez

Research Associate, Hispanic Research Center
Fordham University

ROBERT E. KRIEGER PUBLISHING COMPANY
MALABAR, FLORIDA
1989

18948463
DLC

7-10-95

Original Edition 1989

Printed and Published by
ROBERT E. KRIEGER PUBLISHING CO., INC.
KRIEGER DRIVE
MALABAR, FLORIDA 32950

Library of Congress Cataloging-in-Publication Data

Rogler, Lloyd H. (Lloyd Henry), 1930-
    Hispanics and mental health : a framework for research/Lloyd H.
    Rogler, Robert G. Malgady, Orlando Rodriquez—Original ed.
        p. cm.
    Includes indexes.
    ISBN 0-89464-248-0 (alk. paper)

    1. Hispanic Americans—Mental health. 2. Hispanic Americans—
Mental health services. 3. Hispanic Americans—Mental health
—Research. I. Title.
    [DNLM: 1. Hispanic Americans—psychology. 2. Mental Health.
3. Mental Health Services. 4. Research. WA305 R7345h]
RC451.5.H57R64   1989
362.2′08968073—dc19
DNLM/DLC
for Library of Congress   88-37203
                                                        CIP

10   9   8   7   6   5   4   3   2

CONTENTS

iii

Preface and Acknowledgments

This book presents a conceptual framework which organizes mental health research on Hispanics. Imbedded into the framework is a series of research problems focusing upon mental health issues among Hispanics. These research problems are intended to chart important avenues of research which, if taken, we believe would increase our scientific understanding of mental health and provide a stronger basis for the formulation of mental health policy for Hispanics.

How is the utility of the framework to be assessed? One answer to this question lies in the pages ahead discussing the contributions the framework makes. Another answer lies in the multiple functions the framework already has performed in the life of Fordham University's Hispanic Research Center. Although much of the framework was developed earlier, it was first put into use in response to the import of the political directives of President Ronald Reagan's incoming administration in 1981. The new administration's research agenda severely constricted the National Institute of Mental Health (NIMH) guidelines for psychosocial and cultural research. Since the NIMH was the Center's main sponsor, adaptations had to be made if the Center was to survive. The framework enabled the adaptations and rapidly became the Center's organizing principle. It provided the conceptual basis for research projects which subsequently were funded, internally organized the Center's research efforts, and situated the overall research program in a context of broader concerns. Over the years, it has proven its utilitarian value: to this day it has met the test of changing guidelines of what constitutes mental health relevant research and has withstood the professional scrutiny of numerous mental health researchers.

A preliminary statement of the framework was published in 1983 in the Center's tenth monograph, *A Conceptual Framework for Mental Health Research on Hispanic Populations,* by L.H. Rogler and R.S. Cooney, G. Costantino, B.F. Earley, B. Grossman, D.T. Gurak, R.G. Malgady, O. Rodriguez, with the assistance of K. Colleran, P. Elwell, E. Schroder-Guerrero,

E. Klass and Y. Martinez-Ward. The authors of the present work took this preliminary statement as a point of departure in formulating new sets of research problems at the forefront of mental health research on Hispanics and in developing still further the framework's general contributions. The end result, this book, represents a substantially new statement resting upon a foundation previously established and tested.

A number of persons have assisted in the production of this book. Stasia Madrigal edited successive drafts of the manuscript and constructed the indices. Mercedes Rivera typed several drafts of the manuscript. Elizabeth Ospina contacted agencies and persons to provide us with necessary information. Dharma Cortes checked the accuracy of references to published materials. Giuseppe Costantino's help enabled us to draft the vignettes presented at the beginning of Chapters 2, 3, 4, 5, and 6. We wish to express our appreciation for their valuable contributions.

Portions of Chapter 2 originally appeared in "The Migration Experience and Mental Health: Formulations Relevant to Hispanics and Other Immigrants," by L.H. Rogler, D.T. Gurak, and R.S. Cooney, published in pp. 72-84, *Health and Behavioral Research Agenda for Hispanics,* edited by M. Gaviria and J.D. Arana, Simon Bolivar Research Monograph (No.1), University of Illinois, Chicago. This monograph is in the public domain. Portions of Chapters 3 and 4 originally appeared in the following articles published in the *American Psychologist,* a journal of the American Psychological Association (APA, copyright 1947): "Ethnocultural and Linguistic Bias in Mental Health Evaluation of Hispanics," by R.G. Malgady, L.H. Rogler and G. Costantino, vol. 42, no.3, March 1987; and "What Do Culturally Sensitive Mental Health Services Mean? The Case of Hispanics," by Lloyd H. Rogler, Robert G. Malgady, Giuseppe Costantino and Rena Blumenthal, vol. 42, no. 6, June 1987. Portions of those articles used in this work have been reprinted and adapted by permission of the publisher.

This volume represents the fifteenth monograph produced by the Hispanic Research Center to stimulate interest in Hispanic concerns. The Center was established at Fordham University in 1977, under Grant 2 RO1 MH 30569 from the NIMH, Minority Research Resources Branch, to work toward five major objectives: (1) to develop and conduct policy-relevant epidemiological/clinical services research on Hispanic mental health issues; (2) to increase the small pool of scholars trained in Hispanic mental health research and to upgrade their research skills through the provision of apprenticeship training and other mechanisms; (3) to provide technical assistance to organizations and individuals interested in the mental health problems of Hispanics; (4) to disseminate information on issues relevant to

Hispanic mental health; and (5) to develop a research environment for scholars from the mental health disciplines.

Lloyd H. Rogler
Albert Schweitzer University Professor
in the Humanities
Director, Hispanic Research Center
Fordham University

Chapter 1

Mental Health Research and Hispanics

This book seeks to attain two interrelated objectives. The first is to present a conceptual framework which organizes clinical service mental health research according to a hypothetical temporal sequence composed of five phases. The second is to formulate research problems relevant to Hispanic mental health in each of the five phases of the framework. Throughout the book, we will attempt to interrelate the framework and the research problem in order to provide an overview of important issues and new insights into mental health research on Hispanics. We hope that these contributions will expand our knowledge of the sociocultural and psychological processes affecting the lives of Hispanics and inform public policy and practice designed to improve their well-being. However, first we must ask several basic questions implied by this effort: Why the need for a framework for clinical service mental health research? Why the formulation of a series of research problems? Why focus upon Hispanic populations?

Over a decade has now elapsed since the *Report to the President's Commission on Mental Health* (1978) was issued. The report remarked on the growth of research: over 2000 published items then available on Hispanic mental health, of which 75 percent had been produced in the preceding eight years. The report, however, pointedly criticized the literature on Hispanic mental health research. It noted flaws across the entire spectrum of research procedures, as well as the use of stereotypical explanations of findings and the grave absence of programmatically oriented research. One central flaw noted by the report was the lack of an integrated body of research literature. With the exception of the effort represented by this book, this flaw remains unremedied. True, there have been innumerable listings of priority research topics, usually as a result of the deliberations at research conferences. And there have been occasional schemes proposed for organizing the research literature, usually framed at a level more abstract than the priority listings (NIMH, 1987). But none of these efforts so far has fulfilled the minimal requirement of an effective framework that interrelates categories and is comprehensive in coverage. If the need for such integration was evident a decade ago, today it is of even greater importance as a way of introducing some order into the ever-increasing research on the mental health of Hispanics. Despite such an increase, the research problems to be presented in the following chapters demonstrate that critically important issues affecting the mental health of Hispanics remain unresolved and even unaddressed.

The framework we propose is intuitively simple and understandable. To explain it, let us take the example of a person who has undergone and finished professional treatment for a mental health problem. What were the typical experiences of that person? Earlier, at some time, some combination of factors had produced the person's emotional problem; having experienced the discomfort and pain of the problem, the afflicted person, probably with the assistance of significant others, sought help from some part of the mental health establishment; when such contact was formed, the person's emotional problem was evaluated; some kind of mental health treatment was administered; and after treatment the person was—or was not—relieved of the original problem and returned—or did not return—to an effective level of social functioning.

The framework we propose is a representation of the afflicted person's successive experiences, beginning with the emergence of the emotional problem and ending with the post-treatment period. In the framework, these experiences are temporally arrayed into five phases, each of which encompasses the collective experiences of a large number of persons—in our case, Hispanics—who have undergone the clinical service process. The process is not arbitrarily divided into these five phases; we shall see that significant bodies of mental health research on Hispanics coincide with the five-phase structure.

- Phase One of the framework involves factors contributing to or associated with the emergence of a mental health problem.
- Phase Two designates the intricate help-seeking efforts which may or may not lead the afflicted person to contact official mental health service providers.
- Phase Three focuses upon the attempts, valid or invalid, by such help providers to evaluate or diagnose the client's psychological condition.
- Phase Four begins when official mental health providers attempt to deal with the problem through therapeutic interventions.
- Phase Five involves the termination of treatment and the client's attempted resumption of customary social roles away from the therapeutic setting, whether relieved of the original problem or not.

Thus, in addition to organizing collective experiences into phases, the framework projects the phases forward into a temporal sequence which begins with the rise of emotional problems and ends in the post-treatment period. Because it is prospectively oriented, the framework sensitizes the student of mental health to a variety of issues, perhaps one of the broadest being the untold numbers of persons who drop out of the process which spans the five-phase framework.

Two observations need to be made about the framework. The first already has been implied. The framework does not assume the success of the person's help-seeking effort in allaying the emotional problem which prompted the effort, nor does it predict where the effort will terminate. It is very probable, for example, that many emotional problems, even severe ones, are alleviated or contained without ever reaching professional mental health providers because of the interventions of friends, relatives, religious or grassroot organizations. For example, only about one out of every five persons with a clinical diagnosis of depression had seen a mental health professional in the preceding year (Roberts, 1987). It is probable also that persons may traverse the entire sequence of phases unrelieved of the original emotional problem, or that they may drop out from any one phase only to reenter the clinical service sequence at some time in the future. Thus, the framework does not predict the specific trajectories persons will follow and explicitly allows for the possibility of trajectories signifying repeated patterns of recidivism, of entering and leaving phases of the framework. The uncovering of such trajectories is the appropriate task of research. But it is the use of the framework in research which enables the identification of the trajectories of cohorts of persons in the phases of the clinical service sequence.

The second observation needs to be considered at somewhat greater length because of the need to emphasize an expanded vision of what constitutes mental health relevant research in relation to the framework. We have spoken in terms of the successive experiences of persons afflicted with emotional problems and their trajectories through the framework's sequential phases. Although this focus deals with the proximate experiences of the afflicted person, it in no way obviates or diminishes the need for research oriented toward macro societal and historical forces. We are very much in agreement with Fried's statement (1980) that macro-level forces ". . .have both overt and subtle ramifications that invade every sphere of life" (p.68). One sphere incessantly invaded by such forces is the person's psychological well-being.

To illustrate this observation, we turn briefly to the substantial tradition of research attempting to delineate the intricate connections between economic change and behavioral disorder. The connections have been examined through cross-sectional and longitudinal research based upon data collected at the individual and aggregate level (Dooley and Catalano, 1980). For example, Catalano and Dooley (1977) were able to show through longitudinal research at the aggregate and individual level that economic changes in Kansas City affected the life-event changes of the city's residents which in turn influenced their level of depression. The city's aggregate unemployment rates proved to be the best economic predictor of psychological depression. This type of research shows the longitudinal relation between macro-level forces, life-event changes in the person's immediate environment, and psychological distress. Its pertinence to the framework's first phase, focusing upon the emergence of mental health problems, is immediately evident. In turn, influences converging on the first phase can be expected to stimulate the movement of persons into subsequent phases.

Examples of broader historical changes which can affect the other phases more or less directly also can be provided. Thus, Rogler et al. (1987) have argued that two events converged in the decade of the 60s to focus attention upon the need for culturally sensitive mental health services for economically disadvantaged minority populations. First, the rise of the civil rights movement when blacks and other minority groups insisted that the institutional structure of American society be made more responsive to their needs and less exclusionary of their participation as citizens in a pluralistic democracy. Second was the enactment of President Johnson's Great Society programs and the rapid development of community mental health programs. As these programs expanded to cover new economically disadvantaged catchment areas with populations which never before had received professional mental health care, many of the deficiencies of traditional service systems and therapies became evident. Thus, historically, the insistence upon the need for culturally sensitive minority-oriented mental health services, associated with the community mental health movement, fit into the broader civil rights movement's drive toward rendering institutional structures more responsive to the rights and needs of minority groups.

The historical changes converged upon mental health services for Hispanics in efforts to increase the accessibility of mental health services, an issue imbedded in the second phase of the framework; in raising questions as to the cultural sensitivity of the customary mental health diagnostic procedures and tests, a problem relevant to the third phase; in urging changes in the usual treatments and in the development of culturally appropriate therapeutic interventions, a need evident in Phase Four; and, in the context of the deinstitutionalization movement, by focusing attention upon post-treatment rehabilitation, an issue pertinent to Phase Five. The point is that the processes designated by the framework, although analytically separable from other processes, do not in fact operate in a societal or historical vacuum. They are profoundly influenced by broader macro forces operating at diverse societal levels. For this reason, mental health research must retain an expanded vision of its subject matter. Consistent with such a vision, the framework provides the basis for a definition of mental health relevant research as any research at whatever level which is demonstrably relevant to any one of the five phases, taken either separately or jointly.

Even though we recognize the importance of macro-oriented mental health research, the research problems presented in this book are formulated mostly at the micro level, dealing with factors and events proximate to the lives of persons. Our reason for this is programmatic, not substantive. In an introductory work such as this, it is important to attend first to the viability of the framework in organizing research seeking to explain factors and events immediate to the lives of Hispanics who have come to experience emotional distress. At an elementary level, this would serve to ground the framework in the experiences of persons developing mental health problems, seeking help, being diagnosed and treated, and living their lives after treatment. The formulation of research could then be projected further into the successive experiences of persons traversing the framework's phases. At the same time, a firmer basis would be provided for studies oriented toward the impact of macro forces, for then we would know, with perhaps more clarity and specificity than we now have, what it is in particular that such forces converge upon in the immediate lives of emotionally distressed Hispanics.

Let us provide a brief illustration by means of the concept of acculturation which will be seen to play a major role in Hispanic mental health research. Acculturation refers to the complex process whereby the behaviors and attitudes of a migrant group change toward the dominant group as a result of exposure to a cultural system that is significantly different. This process has immediate experiential meaning in the lives of Hispanics. It means the degree to which they retain the use of Spanish and master and use English, expose themselves to the host society's Spanish or English mass media, develop consumption preferences coinciding with mass culture, accept the terms of a bureaucratically organized society, and other such things. Without foreshadowing the points to be discussed in subsequent chapters, it can be stated that acculturation appears to be relevant to the Hispanics' experiences in each of the framework's five phases, although exactly in which way and under which conditions remain to be uncovered by research. As research proceeds, hopefully, to resolve such ambiguities, the opportunities will become available to trace the impact of macro level forces—such as bilingual educational policies, mass media decisions on the distribution of ethnically oriented television and radio programs or publications, the adaptation of bureaucratic policies and services to the clients' culture, and so on—upon the experiential components of acculturation in the lives of Hispanics traversing the phases of the framework. The program of research which is required is long indeed, but the need for direction in the ever-expanding research effort is clearly evident.

To provide this direction in the context of the five-phase framework, we have chosen as a vehicle the concept of a research problem. Merton's analysis (1959) of this concept in sociological research is satisfactory to our purposes. He argues that the posing of an important originating question or hypothesis in science is a disciplined and difficult activity. Why? Because questions asked at random do not inherently contain the necessary scientific credentials. Rather, such credentials are conferred upon questions by demonstrating systematically that answers to them are consequential in significantly affecting the structure of associated beliefs, in whatever way the effects occur. Were it not for this process, research would be devoid of direction because there would be a theoretically unjustified multiplication of ad hoc questions. This type of significance will be evident in the chapters that follow. However, there is another type of significance, not exclusive of the former, which is customarily found in applied research attempting to contribute to the solution or amelioration of social problems, such as those implicating the experiences of emotionally distressed Hispanics. Here, significance is couched in terms of the research being consequential to social policy or public practice. This type of significance, also to be seen in the chapters which follow, is particularly relevant to research on the lives of disadvantaged minority persons, many of whom are to be found among Hispanics.

The concept of a research problem, therefore, contains the questions to be asked and the rationale for their significance. In actual research, there is a third component, namely the procedures or the research design to be used to answer the questions posed. Research designs, however, can and do vary substantially even when addressing a single significantly posed question. For this reason, decisions pertinent to research design usually are rooted in the specific context of the research project and its setting. Since our effort is aimed at the formulation of general research problems, general methodological problems will be discussed, but specific issues of research design will not be given the extensive attention which would be required in the development of specific research projects.

The choice of research problems as the vehicle means that the purpose here is not a comprehensive review of the literature on Hispanic mental health, even though the proposed framework also lends itself to that purpose. Extensive reviews of this literature are available elsewhere (Padilla and Lindholm, 1983). Such reviews are critically important in providing an overview of the distribution of the research effort, the most commonly used theoretical orientations and research designs, and the most recent findings and conclusions. However, the very rapid growth of the literature on Hispanic mental health soon renders as outdated any single review. Our task, rather, will be to selectively use critically important portions of the literature to formulate research problems likely to endure beyond the findings of specific research projects or reviews. We hope the formulations serve to structure avenues for future research within the context of the five-phase clinical service framework. Vignettes developed from case histories of clients of a community mental health center are presented at the beginning of the chapters discussing the phases. They are reminders that the abstract statements of research problems are rooted in actual human experiences.

Why focus the formulation of research problems on Hispanic populations? To answer this question we begin with some important characteristics of Hispanics. Defined in broad terms, Hispanics are persons who were born in a Spanish-speaking country, including the Commonwealth of Puerto Rico, or who are Hispanic by virtue of parentage or other predecessors. They share a common language, are prevailingly Roman Catholic, and are historically interlinked by their common ties to Spanish colonialism in the New World. In the United States, they comprise the second largest minority group, blacks being the largest. Their growth in numbers resulting from immigration and natural increase exceeds that of any other group in the United States. In 1987 they numbered about 18.8 million, almost a 30 percent increase over the number registered by the U.S. Bureau of the Census in 1980. These numbers do not include the 3.2 million Puerto Ricans living in the Commonwealth of Puerto Rico in 1980 or the unknown number of Hispanics who were not counted due to problems associated with conducting a census on minority populations and undocumented Hispanic immigrants in the United States.

Hispanics vary in their national background, with 60 percent of Mexican origin, 14 percent of Puerto Rican origin, and 7 percent of Cuban origin, the remainder having as their nationality the Spanish-speaking republics of Central and South America and the Caribbean. Thus, the largest three groups—Mexicans, Puerto Ricans, and Cubans—when combined, comprise over 80 percent of the Hispanic population in the United States. Geographically, Hispanics are widely dispersed. Mexican Americans are concentrated in the five southwestern states and in the Midwest; Puerto Ricans in New York, other mid-Atlantic states, and the Midwest; Cuban Americans in Florida and northern New Jersey. The pattern of geographical dispersal at the national level is replicated in local settings. Thus, in New York City and its surrounding area, there are clearly identifiable neighborhoods of Puerto Ricans, Dominicans, Cubans, and Colombians. Hispanics living in the United States are an urban people.

Demographic studies of Hispanics (Gurak and Rogler, 1980) converge upon two related themes: their diversity and the disadvantaged status of some nationality groups comprising this diversity. Hispanics differ markedly in first-generation status: Mexican Americans, 18 percent; Puerto Ricans, 55 percent; and Cubans, 82 percent. (However, in absolute numbers there have been more recent immigrants among Mexican Americans than among the other two groups.) Therefore, there is substantial variability with respect to their proximity to the migration experience. Non-Hispanics in the United States have a median age of about 30.4. Mexican Americans and Puerto Ricans are a young population with median ages about ten years younger than those of non-Hispanics. Cuban Americans, however, are about six years older than non-Hispanics. The disparity in age between the sexes varies in the three groups: about the same among Mexican Americans; Puerto Rican women about 4.4 years older than Puerto Rican men; and Cuban women about 5.6 years older than Cuban men (Gurak, 1981). The age and age-by-sex differences among Hispanics have broad implications for life cycle and family formation experiences. Marriage studies in New York relevant to family formation indicate variability in rates of outgroup marriage: Puerto Ricans marry within their own group at a higher rate than Central Americans and Dominicans. Also, unlike other Hispanic groups, the Puerto Ricans' generational status is not related to their rate of outgroup marriages: they sustain a high rate of ingroup marriage into the second generation (Fitzpatrick and Gurak, 1979). In sum, homogeneity is not the prevailing demographic pattern: Hispanics differ in generational status, age structure, and patterns of endogamous marriage.

The percentage of Hispanics living below the poverty level is significantly higher than for non-Hispanic whites (Hispanic Policy Development Project, 1984) but, consistent with the diversity of Hispanic groups, there are marked differences among them with respect to their educational, occupational, and income characteristics. If, for purposes of brevity, these characteristics are combined into a concept of socioeconomic status, general patterns can be identified. Among Hispanics, Cubans enjoy the advantages of a higher socioeconomic status, followed by Mexican Americans, and then by Puerto Ricans who are at the very bottom of the socioeconomic hierarchy. Two rapidly growing Hispanic groups in New York City are differentially located in this hierarchy: Colombians, a prevailing middle-class group, tending toward the socioeconomic status of Cubans; and Dominicans, above but tending toward the lower socioeconomic level of Puerto Ricans. Levels and types of labor force participation undergird such socioeconomic differences, as do differential educational attainments, but another factor of rapidly emerging importance is the rise of female-headed households, in particular, among Puerto Ricans: in 1980, 44 percent of New York City's Puerto Rican households were headed by women as opposed to 32 percent of such households in the category of "other Hispanics" (Mann and Salvo, 1985). These households have income earnings about one-half those of intact households. The feminization-of-poverty theme applies to much of the Puerto Rican experience in New York City.

As brief as this overview of Hispanics is, it still would be incomplete if the situation of New York City's Puerto Ricans were not to be singled out for further attention. This attention is possible because of Mann and Salvo's detailed comparison (1985) of Puerto Ricans and "other Hispanics" in New York City based upon the 1980 census. In addition to the comparatively high percentage of Puerto Rican households headed by females, there are other differences between Puerto Ricans and "other Hispanics." Thus, in comparison to "other Hispanics" in New York City, Puerto Ricans were younger and less often members of an extended family; they had fewer high school graduates, lower median household incomes, less participation in the labor force, and a greater dependence upon public assistance. To this profile depicting the Puerto Ricans' pervasively rooted social and economic disadvantages should be added the findings of other studies (Gurak, 1981) demonstrating that in New York City the residential segregation of Puerto Ricans from non-Hispanic whites is greater than the segregation experienced by Hispanics in 28 other large urban areas; this finding intertwines with the previously cited pattern of intergenerational persistence in low rates of outgroup marriage among Puerto Ricans. The Puerto Ricans are a socially and economically deprived Hispanic group experiencing substantial structural isolation.

Epidemiological studies indicate that socioeconomic status is inversely related to mental health problems (Schwab and Schwab, 1982). The relationship of such problems to immigration and acculturation, on the other hand, remains a hypothesis which will be discussed in the next chapter. Nonetheless, viewed from such a perspective, the characteristics of Hispanics—in particular, New York City's Puerto Ricans—would suggest a population which is at high risk to the development of mental health problems. It is a high-risk population which is rapidly increasing in size, a trend which converges with the rise and rapid development of the community mental health movement with the proliferation of centers attempting to provide services in previously unserved catchment areas. The complex interactions between the mental health needs of a growing high-risk population and the institutional structures seeking to deliver mental health services to this population make Hispanics a strategically important group upon which to focus the formulation of research problems. It is these interactions which continue to stimulate the research efforts directed at Hispanics, efforts which promise to add to our fund of basic knowledge about mental health problems while seeking to improve the mental health welfare of Hispanics. The formulation of research problems in each of the five phases of the framework proposed here, we believe, introduces conceptual order into this research effort.

References

Catalano, R. and Dooley, D. (1977). Economic predictors of depressed mood and stressful life events in a metropolitan community. *Journal of Health and Social Behavior* 18: 292-307.

Dooley, D. and Catalano, R. (1980). Economic change as a cause of behavioral disorder. *Psychology Bulletin* 87 (3): 450-468.

Fitzpatrick, J.P. and Gurak, D.T. (1979). *Hispanic Intermarriage in New York City: 1975.* Bronx, NY: Hispanic Research Center, Fordham University, Monograph No. 2.

Fried, M. (1980). Stress, strain, and role adaptation: Conceptual issues. In G. Coelho and P. Ahmed (Eds.), *Uprooting and Development,* p. 68. New York: Plenum Press.

Gurak, D.T. (1981). Family structural diversity of Hispanic ethnic groups. *Research Bulletin,* April-July 1981 (vol. 4, nos.2-3), Hispanic Research Center, Fordham University.

Gurak, D.T. and Rogler, L.H. (1980). New York's new immigrants: Who and where they are. The Hispanics. *New York University Education Quarterly,* vol. XI, No. 4, Summer.

Hispanic Policy Development Project (1984). *The Hispanic Almanac.* New York: Author.

Mann, E.S. and Salvo, J.J. (1985). Characteristics of new Hispanic immigrants to New York City: A comparison of Puerto Rican and non-Puerto Rican Hispanics. *Research Bulletin,* January-April (vol.8, nos.1-2), Hispanic Research Center, Fordham University, New York City.

Merton, R.K. (1959). Notes on problem-finding in sociology. In R.K. Merton, L. Broom, and L.S. Cottrell, Jr. (Eds.), *Sociology Today.* New York: Basic Books.

Minority Mental Health Services Research Conference Proceedings (August 1987), Minority Research Resources Branch, Division of Biometry and Applied Sciences, National Institute of Mental Health.

Padilla, A. and Lindholm, K. (1983). Hispanic Americans: Future behavioral science research directions. In National Institute of Mental Health (Ed.), *Behavioral Sciences Research in Mental Health: An Assessment of the State of the Science and Recommendations for Research Directions,* vol. II, pp. XXV 1-32. Washington, D.C.: NIMH.

Roberts, R. (1987). Epidemiological issues in measuring preventive effects. In R.F. Muños (Ed.), *Depression Prevention: Research Directions.* New York: Hemisphere Publishing.

Rogler, L.H., Malgady, R.G., Costantino, G. and Blumenthal, R. (1987). What do culturally sensitive mental health services mean? The case of Hispanics. *American Psychologist* 42 (6): 565-570.

Schwab, J.J. and Schwab, M.E. (1982). *Sociocultural Roots of Mental Illness: An Epidemiologic Survey.* New York: Plenum Medical Book Co., 2nd printing.

Special Populations Sub-Task Panel on Mental Health of Hispanic Americans (1978). *Report to the President's Commission on Mental Health.* Los Angeles: Spanish-Speaking Mental Health Research Center, University of California, p. 4.

Chapter 2

Phase One: Emergence of Mental Health Problems

With only one year of schooling and no knowledge of English, Mr. José Cintrón—cutter of sugar cane in the fields of Puerto Rico—was in need of help when he arrived in New York City. His sisters helped him, but it was his god-daughter and her husband who first gave him room and board in their own apartment, then found him a good job and his own apartment in the same building. As a kitchen helper in a private club, washing dishes and making juice, he was given three meals a day and could earn up to $100 a week with overtime. Everything at work went well for six years but then the club hired a new chief cook. Even though the cook was Hispanic, he repeatedly criticized Mr. Cintrón for not speaking English. The cook spoke to the other kitchen helpers in English, cutting Mr. Cintrón out of their daily conversations. Mr. Cintrón began to feel nervous and anxious. He felt they were talking about him. One of the helpers began to accuse Mr. Cintrón of stealing soap, brillo pads, and other kitchen supplies. One afternoon, after receiving his weekly pay and ready to go on Christmas vacation, he was ordered by the the chief cook to stay at work. Mr. Cintrón exploded in anger, told the cook he could no longer take the abuse, and resigned.

Nonetheless, he decided to enjoy his vacation, and went shopping that night for Christmas gifts for his relatives. Returning to his apartment in the South Bronx, which recently had been burglarized twice, two men accosted him, took his wallet, then stabbed him repeatedly. He crawled to his god-daughter's apartment on the second floor and was taken to the hospital in critical condition. Three weeks later he was released. Mr. Cintrón was now terrified at the prospect of leaving his apartment, but with the help of his god-daughter's husband, he was able to return to his old job. But his coworkers began to speak in English once again, he thought, to gossip about him. He quit the job and found the name of a doctor in a Spanish newspaper. The doctor gave him pills and told him he was suffering from "mental depression."

* * *

Phase One research focuses upon factors that lead to the development and manifestation of mental health problems. The approaches to the study of mental health problems can be as varied as the diverse methodologies used to study the etiologic factors of mental illness. We make the assumption, however, that when information is sparse, the approach used should be broadly delineated in scope in order to cover a diversity of sociocultural and economic factors. Thus, psychiatric epidemiology is the indicated method in this phase of the framework.

Findings from psychiatric epidemiology pose questions about the comparative distribution of mental health problems in Hispanic and other populations. Answers to such questions provide clues to the etiology of mental distress and a baseline for estimating the extent to which a population utilizes mental health resources, as we shall see in the next chapter. These questions are also important to the future direction of Hispanic mental health care, since proponents of increased and more culturally sensitive mental health services for Hispanics premise their arguments on the assumption that the mental health needs of Hispanics are both disproportionately high and underserved. Thus, our first research problem in this phase of the framework focuses on the distribution of mental health problems among Hispanics. Although this research question seems elementary, the answers which have been provided by epidemiological studies are by no means consistent. Consequently, we shall attempt to distinguish between one group of studies that suggest that Hispanics evidence higher prevalence rates of mental disorder compared to other ethnic populations and another group of studies suggesting that they do not. We will note methodological weaknesses in the psychiatric epidemiology literature in both camps, as well as directions for future research.

Since a large number of Hispanics are first-generation immigrants and have experienced fundamental changes in their sociocultural environments, our second research problem in this phase focuses on an old but essentially unanswered question: Does the migration experience create mental distress? If so, under what conditions? We will attempt to develop the outlines of a conceptual approach, inferentially based on mental health research, as provisional answers to these questions and as a basis for future research.

The third and last research problem in this phase focuses upon the stress process as experienced by Hispanics. This problem can be looked at both as part of the migration process and separately outside the context of migration. As formulated in epidemiological research, the stress process involves the complex interactions between stressful life events, the emergence of mental health problems, and factors which act as mediators between the emergence of stress and the appearance of mental distress. Much of the rapidly growing literature on the stress process has historical roots in epidemiological research suggesting that economically disadvantaged, marginated groups experience more mental health problems than groups in the mainstream of society. Since large segments of the Hispanic population can be characterized as disadvantaged and marginated, the examination of the stress process experienced by Hispanics is consistent with the history of previous research.

The Comparative Distribution of Mental Health Problems

Arguments that Hispanics experience more mental health problems than other ethnic populations are based partly on psychiatric epidemiology research indicating that populations with the demographic, socioeconomic, and experiential characteristics of Hispanics have comparatively higher rates of mental illness. For example, the finding of the well-known study by Hollingshead and Redlich (1958) which confirmed an inverse relationship between socioeconomic status and some forms of treated mental illness has been generalized to the situation of Hispanics (Rogler et al., 1983). The replication of Hollingshead and Redlich's finding in a variety of settings, and in reference to the association between low socioeconomic status and prevalence of schizophrenia (Dohrenwend, 1966), strengthens the inference to the case of Hispanics. The typically disadvantaged socioeconomic characteristics of Hispanics, particularly Mexican Americans and Puerto Ricans, render them vulnerable to mental health disorders.

Similarly, there is a long history of research which relates the migration experience to mental health, most of which is based upon hospital admission or treatment records of immigrants versus non-immigrants. This research has implicated the migration experience in mental illness across a variety of ethnic groups, including native- and foreign-born whites, blacks, and Hispanics, in cross-sections of American society (e.g., Odegaard, 1932; Malzberg, 1962; Lee, 1963; Kleiner and Parker, 1959). However, this research exhibits widely recognized methodological problems commonly associated with the study of self-selected institutionalized populations and related to the introduction of appropriate controls in comparisons between migrants and non-migrants (Sanua, 1970); the operational specification of the concepts of immigrant and migration (e.g., Kleiner and Parker, 1965; Parker et al., 1969); the analysis of undifferentiated categories of "all mental disorders" (Kleiner and Parker, 1965); and the global diagnostic categories (e.g., schizophrenia) subject to unknown margins of diagnostic error (e.g., Jaco, 1960). Whatever the methodological shortcomings of such research, there are reasons for believing, as we shall see presently, that there is a relationship between the components of the migration experience and the onset of mental distress.

Thus, the magnitude of Hispanics' mental health problems has been inferred from their socioeconomic and migratory experiences. Although such inferences do not represent externally valid generalizations, they are not entirely speculative. Rather, they are an integral part of the circumstantial evidence supporting the need for carefully designed epidemiological studies to determine the mental health status of Hispanics, either by measuring symptomatology or by classifying individuals according to diagnostic categories of mental disorder, i.e., those listed in the *Diagnostic and Statistical Manual-III* (DSM-III). Unfortunately, the need for sound epidemiological research has not been entirely fulfilled and, for this reason, it constitutes our first research problem. Many of the conclusions of past epidemiological research have been equivocal and, in many instances, hindered by methodological and sampling problems. We will first consider studies reporting higher rates of mental illness among Hispanic populations.

In his review of the literature, Roberts (1980) identified only three papers reporting population-based data on the prevalence of psychological disorders among Mexican Americans. Findings on the comparative distress of Mexican Americans and other ethnic groups have been mixed. However, Roberts' own study in California suggests that ". . .the prevalence of psychological distress among Chicanos is at least as high as in the overall population and, in some respects, higher" (p. 141).

An early study by Srole et al. (1962) found that about half of the 27 Puerto Ricans in the New York sample were diagnosed as having severe or incapacitating symptoms—double the rate for any other ethnic group. However, this study has been criticized because of the limited generalizability of such a small sample size, and because the differential indications of mental illness may have been due to a bias in research methodology and to cultural differences in reporting symptoms (Dohrenwend, 1966).

In a survey of more than 1000 residents of New York City, Dohrenwend and Dohrenwend (1969) found that Puerto Ricans reported significantly greater numbers of psychiatric symptoms than their social-class counterparts in other ethnic groups. The Dohrenwends cautioned that some of the observed differences between ethnic groups may have been due to factors such as cultural differences in response styles, language used to express psychological distress, and different cultural connotations of socially desirable behavior. Haberman's (1976) field studies found that Puerto Ricans in New York City reported even more psychiatric symptoms than island Puerto Ricans, but the root issues of response style, language, and cultural context have remained unresolved.

Other studies have attended to treated prevalence rates of psychological disorder or what is currently termed "rates-under-treatment" (Schwab and Schwab, 1978). Comparing a non-minority group and a global group of minority patients, Gross et al. (1969) found higher prevalence rates for the minority population. Ethnic minority patients were more likely to be diagnosed as schizophrenic and then treated in a psychiatric emergency room than were non-minority patients who tended to be more often classified as neurotic and referred to outpatient psychiatric services. More recently, Baskin et al. (1981) reported similar findings comparing blacks and Hispanics with whites at large community mental health centers and psychiatric hospitals.

The epidemiological literature on Mexican Americans is also inconclusive. For example, Vega et al. (1985) cited some of the conflicting findings of Mexican American prevalence rates and, in a study of farm workers, concluded that this population experiences such a high level of psychiatric symptomatology as to be at "extraordinary risk." Other recent surveys of untreated populations of Mexican Americans are in substantial agreement with this position, based on the assessment of depressive symptomatology (Vega et al., 1984) and psychiatric symptoms and dysfunction in general (Warheit et al., 1985).

We now turn to studies reporting lower rates of mental illness or no difference between rates for the Hispanic population. Some early research by Jaco (1960) found that Mexican Americans had lower prevalence rates under treatment than non-Hispanics. In a recent study of true prevalence rates based on probability samples of Mexican Americans and non-Hispanic whites, Karno et al. (1987) reported findings essentially consistent with Jaco's earlier work. The Karno et al. study was a carefully designed sampling of over 3000 households in the Los Angeles area (with a response completion rate of 68 percent) in which the Diagnostic Interview Schedule (DIS) was administered to elicit symptoms indicative of 40 DSM-III mental disorders. The major findings indicated relatively similar prevalence rates for Mexican Americans and non-Hispanic whites on most diagnostic categories, with the exceptions of substance abuse, cognitive impairment, and depression. Non-Hispanic whites had higher drug abuse rates than Mexican Americans, while the reverse was true for alcohol abuse. Karno et al. attributed these differences largely to socioeconomic factors; namely, that the lower socioeconomic status Mexican Americans turn to alcohol as a less expensive outlet than drugs. Mexican Americans were found to be substantially more cognitively impaired than non-Hispanic whites, but this was attributed to cultural differences, language difficulties, and their lower educational attainment. Similarly, although non-Hispanic white females had the highest rate of depression, this was highly correlated with, and presumably a function of, their greater drug abuse. However, we question why higher rates of alcohol abuse among Mexican Americans similarly would not lead to greater depression.

Although the Karno et al. study is based on a sizeable and carefully selected sample, it is not without its shortcomings. The true prevalence rates reported in this study were based upon six-month and lifetime prevalence reports, the latter being a highly questionable technique in terms of validity of retrospective self-reports across the life span. Further, as Karno et al. acknowledge, the Diagnostic Interview Schedule omits the great majority of mental disorders enumerated in the DSM-III; thus, many extant psychological diagnoses within the sample of respondents may have been overlooked. Finally, Karno et al. speculate that non-respondents, who constituted 32 percent of the households contacted, probably included a larger proportion of persons with mental disorders than those who consented to be interviewed.

Tangential to the theme of comparing Hispanics to non-Hispanics, a study of different Hispanic populations compared Mexican Americans in the southwest United States, Cuban Americans in Florida, and Puerto Ricans in New York (Moscicki et al., 1987). What is of interest in this study is that the prevalence of depression, reported without a non-Hispanic comparison group, was consistent with the prevalence rates reported on Mexican Americans by Karno et al. (1987), but only for Mexican Americans and Cuban Americans. The rate of depression among Puerto Ricans was more than double the rates of the two other Hispanic populations.

Another recent study utilizing a methodology and large-scale sampling procedures similar to the Karno et al. study was conducted by Canino et al. (1987a). The Diagnostic Interview Schedule was used in interviews with over 1000 households in Puerto Rico, with a completion rate of 91 percent, in order to classify individuals according to DSM-III criteria, including criteria for alcohol abuse/dependence. Although no direct comparison was made between native Puerto Ricans and other ethnic groups, prevalence rates were compared with age cohort groups sampled from the general population in New Haven, Baltimore, and St. Louis. At the cohort sites, alcoholism prevalence peaked in the 25 to 44 year-old group and then decreased, while in Puerto Rico alcoholism prevalence increased steadily with age. In the 45 to 64 year-old group, six-month prevalence of alcoholism was nearly three times higher in Puerto Rico than in the New Haven and St. Louis sites, and about 22 percent higher than in the Baltimore site.

The studies reviewed thus far represent a sample of the epidemiological literature related to Hispanic mental health over the past two decades. There are difficult problems in reconciling the equivocal findings of these studies because of the variability of the methodologies employed. Some are based on true prevalence rates and others, on rates-under-treatment. In addition, true prevalence studies vary with respect to type of prevalence rate—point, six-month, or lifetime. Studies of Mexican American as opposed to Puerto Rican populations have yielded discrepancies as well. Enumeration of symptoms versus frequency of categorical diagnoses (symptom clusters) and large versus small sample size are additional sources of variability among studies. Such incongruence between studies renders any attempt at a broad synthesis of research findings virtually impossible.

The development and psychometric refinement of the Diagnostic Interview Schedule (Eaton and Kessler, 1985) and its recent translation into Spanish for the study of indigenous Puerto Rican prevalence rates (Canino et al., 1987b) represent encouraging progress toward the goal of achieving a reliable and valid structured interview that provides DSM-III diagnostic classifications of mental disorder. However, given the limited scope of the diagnoses derived from the interview schedule, at the present time we must conclude that we do not have a comprehensive picture of the relative distributions of DSM-III categories in different ethnic populations. The current trend seems to be that studies employing the Diagnostic Interview Schedule tend to report similar prevalence rates for a circumscribed number of DSM-III diagnoses among Hispanics and non-Hispanic whites, while much of the impetus for believing that mental disorder is more common within Hispanic populations comes from reports of psychiatric symptoms. Canino et al. (1987c) make the insightful comment that more symptoms do not necessarily imply higher rates of mental illness, since the configuration of symptoms, and not the number of symptoms, is linked to diagnostic classification. Thus, it may well be that the conclusions of both camps of studies are correct: Hispanics may indeed report more psychiatric symptoms, yet they may also evidence DSM-III prevalence rates (or clusters of symptoms) which are similar to those of other ethnic groups. This interpretation of the discrepancy among epidemiological studies is purely speculative, but it invites research employing both methodologies—a symptom checklist and structured interview schedule—administered to probability samples of Hispanics and non-Hispanic whites for confirmation.

A similar observation was made by Roberts (1987), who noted that studies of prevalence of mental health problems within the Mexican American population have relied on two strategies: clinical diagnosis and scales or symptom checklists that measure non-clinical impairment. In his review of research using both strategies, viz., the NIMH Center for Epidemiological Studies Depression Scale (CES-D) and the Diagnostic Interview Schedule (DIS), Roberts reported that prevalence data were markedly affected by the order of administration of the scale and interview. When the CES-D followed the DIS, prevalence rates of depression were half the rates obtained when the scale was administered alone or before the DIS. Evidence also suggested that a second administration of the CES-D and the DIS greatly impaired their reliability. The implication of this finding is that the reliability of incidence rates, defined as the difference between two prevalence rates estimated at separate times, must be less than the reliability of either prevalence rate. Roberts also questioned the validity of the DIS, based on previous research reporting low-to-modest concordance between DIS-generated diagnoses and diagnoses rendered by psychiatrists.

Roberts concluded that we still know very little about the epidemiology of psychological disorders in the Mexican American population, based on the studies using either research strategy. He attributed this gap in knowledge to both the lack of epidemiological studies and the inadequacy and incomparability of research that has been completed. He recommended studies of biological and psychosocial risk factors, the latter to be focused on social status, personal resources, life stress, and family history, with an attempt made to partition risk attributable to the unique and joint effects of each source. Research should be based on large national samples, Roberts concluded, with non-Hispanic comparison groups included, and with the longitudinal perspective of incidence studies rather than the cross-sectional prevalence designs. He also supported the need for data collected by both research strategies—clinical diagnosis and level of symptomatology.

One major concern in attempting to make sense of the epidemiology literature is the underlying issue of measurement error, or the way in which factors accompanying the measurement of mental disorder—but conceptually extraneous to mental illness—intrude upon the observed assessment. For example, the assessment of mental health is biased by the extent to which respondents of one cultural group or another are acquiescent or over-compliant in answering questions pertaining to their mental health, or perhaps see the items composing a psychological instrument or interview as reflecting varying degrees of social desirability. The extent to which some behaviors, represented as items on a psychological instrument or questions in an interview, are perceived as characteristically pathological in one culture but not another, or are misunderstood because of the examinee's educational deficits, also distorts the measurement of psychopathology. This issue of measurement bias and accuracy of psychodiagnosis will be discussed in greater detail in Chapter 4 dealing with the third phase of the conceptual framework—the evaluation of mental health status.

A second major issue which pervades the epidemiological literature is whether mental health disorders are estimated from "true" or "under-treatment" prevalence rates. The relationship between the two rates varies depending upon the impediments which separate minority groups from the official mental health service system. Statistics based upon the records of treatment facilities represent the outcome of complex community-based social, psychological, and cultural processes, and more than likely do not have a stable correlation with true prevalence rates across diverse socioeconomic and cultural groups in the population at large. Were under-treatment statistics to be taken as a proxy for true mental disorder rates—thus disregarding the processes separating the two—biases would intrude into the effort to understand Hispanic mental health needs. True prevalence rates of mental health symptoms or disorders must be kept analytically distinct from clinic admission rates, rates of specific diagnostic categories of treated disorders, and rates of utilization of mental health facilities. To confuse these statistics leads to error in estimation of a population's mental health needs, false clues about etiology, and possible misjudgments in setting mental health priorities and policies.

Since both rates reflect the existence of mental health problems, the need now is to move beyond the distinction between true and under-treatment prevalence rates as a dichotomy and toward studies which account for both types of rates. This should enhance our capacity to develop sensitive hypotheses about etiology and to guide mental health service priorities and policies. Toward this end, it is by no means premature to suggest the need for incidence-based rates, or the rates of appearance of mental health problems in a specified period of time, as a way of identifying the sociocultural experiences of Hispanics likely to generate mental health problems.

From the epidemiological literature considered thus far, we can conclude that Hispanics present a profile of demographic characteristics that are associated with increased risk of mental disorder. Inferentially, we would expect Hispanics to display higher prevalence (and incidence) of specific diagnoses and general levels of symptomatology. The literature is inconclusive, for the variety of reasons already mentioned. The trend seems to be that studies employing scales or symptom checklists tend to report greater dis-

tress among Hispanic populations, while the very few studies making diagnostic comparisons report similar prevalence rates across ethnic groups.
Should future studies show similar diagnostic prevalence rates, the following question would demand attention: Why aren't the stresses and symptoms being converted into mental disorders at a rate which would be expected from the high-risk demographic profile of Hispanics?

Although this first phase of the framework temporally precedes the subsequent phases, clearly estimates of the Hispanic population's mental health
status are predicated on the cross-cultural validity of diagnostic and assessment techniques. Thus, while the statistical precision and sophistication of
the epidemiological literature have been increasing in recent years—moving
toward large sample sizes and representatively selected probability samples
from multiple geographic areas—the ultimate credibility of such efforts
rests upon the validity of indicators of mental health status and the diagnoses rendered. It is tempting to argue that Phase One research is a priority
in the framework because of the reverberations Phase One processes create
in the subsequent phases. But the progress which needs to be made in this
phase closely depends upon the development of new and the adaptation of
old psychometric technology in considering how, among Hispanics, cultural and socioeconomic factors influence clinical assessments of mental health
problems.

The Migration Experience and Mental Health

While working on a program of comparative field studies focusing on
the impact of migration on mental health in the New York City area, we
began with a customary review of the literature on the topic and were im-
pressed with the expansive list of variables implicated in the process of migration and adaptation to a new culture. One point became evident: since
migration from one sociocultural system to another implies a radical change
in the environment impinging upon the immigrant, and since social science
represents an effort to understand the products of the interaction between
person and environment, social scientists from a variety of disciplines have
multiplied the number of variables thought to underlie the relationship between migration and mental health. The literature presents enumerations
of variables hypothesized to affect processes connecting migration to mental
distress, much in the manner of a grocery list. We concur with one theme
underlying critical reviews of the literature on migration and mental
health—the need to refocus our attention away from lengthy lists of variables and toward interrelating the complex processes enmeshing the migra-

tion experience and the emergence of mental health problems (see, for example, Murphy, 1973; Verdonk, 1979). The intricacies of the migration process itself challenge the development of new theoretical formulations that will begin to unravel how stressful experiences accompanying migration encroach upon mental health.

The presentation of our second research problem draws from recent theoretical formulations proposed by Rogler et al. (1987). The formulations identify three major sources of stress in the migration experience: insertion into the host society's socioeconomic system, typically at the lower levels of social strata; disturbances in the primary-group interpersonal bonds enmeshing the migrant; and acculturative problems in relation to the host society's culture. These primary sources of stress are analogous to what Pearlin et al. (1981) describe as "role strains" which are deep and personally enveloping, persistent aspects of stress, shaping broad segments of an immigrant's life.

Migration from one culture to another inevitably inserts the person into the host society's socioeconomic system. Immigrants, therefore, are rendered vulnerable to varying degrees of primary strain depending on their position in the socioeconomic system. Most Hispanics are economically disadvantaged, as documented in the first chapter. The stressfulness of lower socioeconomic position is compounded by pressures stemming from fluctuations in the economy, such as changes in inflationary and employment rates which disproportionately impact on those of lower socioeconomic status, and often by the pressures associated with the experience of downward mobility (e.g., Rogg and Cooney, 1980). A common finding is that the occupations of immigrants immediately after migration represent a step down from the jobs they had left in their own country. Thus, in examining the migration experience of Hispanics, attention must be given to the environmental pressures which result from their insertion at the bottom of the socioeconomic ladder, the severe impact of economic fluctuations on their management of daily maintenance, and downward occupational mobility.

This emphasis on economic factors attending the migration experience reflects a trend in the literature. For example, Dooley and Catalano (1980) conducted an analysis of 31 studies examining the relationship between economic change and psychological disorder by classifying the research on two dimensions: cross-sectional versus longitudinal perspectives and individual versus aggregate unit of data analysis. These two dimensions reflect the temporal ordering of the variables and whether the economic change can be directly linked to behavioral disorder in the individual. Based upon a variety of economic labor force measures, such as unemployment rates, and a variety of measures of psychological disorder, such as depression, suicide rates, and mental hospital admissions, Dooley and Catalano confirmed the pervasive importance of economic factors in psychological disorder.

Our discussion of migration-induced stress associated with socioeconomic status also acknowledges a consistent finding in psychiatric epidemiological research—the negative correlation between socioeconomic status and likelihood of psychological disorder. A host of studies conducted in North America and Europe show that, when all types of psychopathology are classified into one group, the rate of disorders in the lowest socioeconomic levels is about two and a half times the rate in the highest levels (Dohrenwend et al., 1980). This pattern of relationship extends beyond diagnostic categories of mental disorder to include specific dimensions of mental health, such as anxiety, depression, and self-esteem, which are the most frequent problems presented by Hispanics at community mental health clinics (Reubens, 1980).

The prevailing but not exclusive interpretation of the negative correlation between socioeconomic status and psychological disorder is that stressful experiences are more intensely concentrated at the bottom of the socioeconomic ladder. Since immigrants tend to enter the host society at lower socioeconomic levels, they experience greater stress relative to their higher positioned socioeconomic counterparts. However, the insertion of immigrant Hispanics at the bottom of society is not invariant; immigrating professionals may experience little or no socioeconomic change, or only temporary status declines. Studies seeking to examine the influence of migration-induced stress on mental health should not always assume downward mobility or low socioeconomic status. Rather, the impact of economic experiences on the emergence of mental health problems should be examined after the immigrant's location in the stratification system has been determined.

This suggestion is illustrated by a study, mentioned in Chapter 1 and conducted by Catalano and Dooley (1977), who longitudinally examined the relationship between economic change at an aggregate level and the experience of life-change events and depression in a probability sample in Kansas City. Their findings indicated that economic changes in the city, especially the unemployment rate, affected life-event changes which, in turn, increased the level of depression of individuals. This study supports the use of both aggregate and individual data in understanding the deleterious impact of environmental forces on life events and everyday distress. We repeat Fried's (1980) statement presented in Chapter 1, that macro societal forces have ". . .overt and subtle ramifications that invade every sphere of life" (p.68).

Despite the prominence of the stress concept as the means of bridging the relationship between socioeconomic status and psychological disorder, an ancillary hypothesis has been suggested by Kessler (1979) and Kessler and Cleary (1980). The work of Kessler is based upon the proposition that individuals vary in their response to stress. Individuals at the lower socioeconomic levels may experience both a disproportionate amount of stress and be more affected by that stress than others at higher socioeconomic levels. The development of this argument has prompted a look at socioeconomic differences in intrapsychic and social resources for coping with stress—a theme in current thinking is that there are fewer resources for coping with stress in the lower socioeconomic settings. This notion will be examined in the next chapter dealing with Hispanic patterns of utilization of traditional, non-traditional, and family support networks.

The second migration-induced primary strain results from the rupturing of the immigrant's supportive interpersonal bonds. The general mental health relevance of such bonds has drawn the attention of a large number of recent studies in psychiatric epidemiology. The pattern of findings which has emerged suggests that the strength of supportive primary group networks is inversely related to psychological distress—when the networks are weakened or attenuated, the probability of psychological distress increases (Aneshensel and Frerichs, 1982; Aneshensel and Stone, 1982; Bell et al., 1982; Billings and Moos, 1985; Bromet et al., 1982). The inverse relationship remains stable even though the measures of support networks and psychological distress vary across studies. Explanations of the relationship conceive of supportive networks as buffers from encroaching stresses and as directly improving mental health.

Whatever explanations eventually prevail, such findings are patently relevant to the migration experience. The underlying supposition is that the interpersonal, supportive bonds left behind by the migrant in the society of origin are not likely to be readily or fully restored in the host society. This interpersonal void reflects the "uprooting" theme ever present in historical accounts of migration to the United States. Despite this common cultural perception, it is instructive to turn to sociological theory to understand the effects of interpersonal bonds on psychological well-being. Modern sociology informs us that psychological functioning is incessantly influenced by membership in primary groups, such as the immediate family or extended family, composed of a circle of persons engaged in intimate face-to-face interpersonal interactions. Durkheim's well-known formulation (1951) that psychic unity is a function of group cohesion has implications for the case of Hispanics—psychological unity or well-being is impaired when migration erodes the bonds of primary groups.

The feeling of loss of group cohesion by Hispanic immigrants is illustrated in a study by Rogler (1984) of first-generation Puerto Ricans in an American city with the fictitious name of Maplewood. The immigrants were asked to evaluate selected aspects of daily life in Maplewood as compared to their native Puerto Rico. Employment conditions, opportunities for children, health care and schooling resources—all reasons for the motivation to migrate from Puerto Rico—were evaluated as better in Maplewood. However, Maplewood was rated substantially worse than Puerto Rico in terms of entertainment, way of life, neighborhood relationships, and friendships. Among those immigrants who reported missing Puerto Rico (90 percent), 60 percent missed their relatives and 18 percent missed their friends. A study by Gurak and Kritz (1984) echoes these common feelings, but this time among Dominicans and Colombians in New York City. Apart from economic improvement, a very strong motive for their migration was family reunification. The strength of the motive toward family reunification is indicative of the stress felt at the loss of contacts with relatives who had migrated earlier. This same pattern of findings may well apply to the motivations associated with the "reverse migration" of Puerto Ricans returning to their homeland. A primary strain, we believe, accompanies the migration-induced disassembly and attempted reassembly of primary group supportive networks.

Migration-induced primary strains based upon position in the socioeconomic system and disruption of primary interpersonal networks are social structural dimensions at the nexus of the migration and mental health linkage. However, a major non-structural dimension should also be considered—the acculturation process. Acculturation refers to the complex process whereby the behaviors and attitudes of the immigrant change toward those of the host society as a result of exposure to the latter's cultural system (Rogler et al., 1983). Although the literature postulates a variety of components of acculturation, those mentioned most frequently are language familiarity and usage, cultural heritage, ethnic pride, interethnic distance, and perceived discrimination (Padilla, 1980).

The acculturative problems of immigrants have long been thought to be stress-inducing. Since such problems are multiple, relatively enduring, and envelop broad segments of the immigrant's life, they can reasonably be thought to comprise—when taken together—a migration-induced primary strain. It is this perception of strain which appears to underlie the increasing number of studies which have sought to test the relationship between acculturation and psychological distress. The studies have produced findings that are strikingly different. Some support the hypothesis that as acculturation to the host society increases, psychological stress is less likely (Torres-Matrullo, 1976; Warheit et al., 1985). Other studies support the hypothesis that blending together the cultures of the society of origin with that of the host society, or some form of biculturalism, is conducive to mental health (Ortiz and Arce, 1984; Szapocznik et al. 1980). Still others have even supported the hypothesis of a positive relationship between acculturation and psychological distress (Burnam et al., 1987). Since these studies vary in so many respects—substantively as well as methodologically—it is difficult to account for the source of such disparate findings.

There is, thus, a need to introduce some conceptual order into the issue to avoid an ever-increasing chaos of contradictory findings. Two recommendations are offered, the first substantive, the second methodological. First, there is a need for the development of theoretical rationales that link acculturation to psychological distress. The absence of such rationales in the conduct of research prevents empirically based findings from challenging theoretical explanations.

As a first step toward this goal, an explanation of the finding of an inverse relationship between acculturation and psychological distress could begin with the idea that isolation from the broad cultural parameters of the host society creates a primary strain. The strain results from living in an unfamiliar, unpredictable world, which impinges upon everyday life but which is not controllable. Acculturation along dimensions involving the acquisition of instrumental skills, such as mastery of English, begins to remove the primary strain: as the unfamiliar world becomes more familiar, it becomes more controllable.

On the other hand, a plausible explanation could be proposed for believing that as acculturation proceeds, especially at an accelerated rate, primary strains associated with psychological and interpersonal changes emerge. The rapid psychic internalization of cultural elements from the host society, such as a normative system prejudicial toward Hispanics, may weaken the immigrant's ego functions and self-concept. In interpersonal contexts, it may sever or weaken the immigrant's supportive familial and communal bonds, and remove the immigrant from traditional sources of nurturance. Thus, primary strains arise from the convergence of both processes, one psychological, the other interpersonal. Independent of such processes, there is the possibility of increasing dysfunctional behaviors with increasing acculturation as a result of the increased learning of the host society's sociocultural environment, as evidenced by Burnam et al.'s (1987) findings that the more acculturated Mexican Americans in Los Angeles have more alcohol and drug dependence.

When the explanations are brought together, it is the bicultural hypothesis, discussed earlier, which appears to us to be the most plausible even in the face of discrepant findings. This hypothesis implies the functionality of an optimal balance in retaining traditional elements while incorporating new ones, with primary strains tending to occur at both extremes away from the balance point in the incorporation of the two cultures. This formulation does not actually contradict those studies showing an inverse relationship between acculturation and psychological distress. While it is true that the measures of acculturation in the studies point toward the degree of acculturation into the host culture, they do not imply that the Hispanic scoring high on acculturation has shed important elements of the native culture. The retention of such elements may actually undergird the immigrant's mental health throughout the experience of increasing acculturation. Rogler and Cooney's (1984) study of intergenerationally linked Puerto Rican families in New York City did not test this formulation, but the findings are consistent with it: the younger adult families in the study attained phenomenal success in their upward mobility, far outdistancing their first-generation parents, but retained a strong bicultural identity.

The second recommendation, methodological in character, is to develop acceptable measures of acculturation. A number of efforts have been made to develop measurement scales of acculturation (Cuellar et al., 1980; Marin et al., 1987; Padilla, 1980; Szapocznik et al., 1978) and some of the efforts have addressed the psychometric problems associated with such scales. But difficult questions still remain to be answered as to whether or not the scales fulfill essential psychometric criteria: various forms of reliability, criterion-related validity, and construct validity. Other questions immediately challenge how the concept of acculturation is itself formulated, and the adequacy of the scales in conjoining the nuances of Hispanic diversity to the cultural context of the host society. Adequate tests of the linkage between acculturation and mental health presuppose clear answers to such questions, in the very same way in which they presuppose adequate psychometric properties in measures of mental health. The pattern of inconsistent findings relevant to the question of the relationship between acculturation and mental health is likely to continue in future research unless serious efforts are made to address the psychometric issues of acculturation scales. We want to emphasize the critical need to undertake systematic, psychometrically oriented research on acculturation scales. The importance of the concept of acculturation is not, as we shall see, limited to the issue being discussed; its importance transcends the five phases of our organizing framework.

We have seen that the second research problem focuses upon migration-induced changes affecting the person's socioeconomic position, interpersonal networks, and acculturative adaptations. We have argued that the specific patterning of such changes imposes upon the immigrant deep, persistent, and enveloping primary strains. Research deriving from this formulation would seek to examine the joint and separate effects of such changes upon the immigrant's mental health status and probe for mediating factors in the relationships which are uncovered. By definition, the changes to be examined apply only to first-generation immigrants who have been extracted from one sociocultural system and inserted into another.

However, one final observation needs to be made. An abundance of research—some of which has already been cited—documents the relationship of socioeconomic status and primary group networks to mental health status among persons who have not experienced change from one sociocultural system to another. In fact, it was such evidence that led us to choose these components to formulate ideas pertaining to the dynamics of migration-induced primary strains. Also, it is likely that the concept of acculturation retains significance in shaping the behavior of second-generation persons, the offspring of immigrants, or even of subsequent generations, as Rogler and Cooney's (1984) intergenerational study of Puerto Rican families suggests. The three strains, in and of themselves, are not uniquely linked to the migration experience, although the experience itself provides the opportunity for examining the impact of socioeconomic, interpersonal network, and acculturative changes upon mental health.

The Stress Process

The third research problem concerns the stress process and Hispanic populations. Intervening between migration-induced primary strains and the emergence of psychological distress are mediating experiences which shape the adaptiveness of the immigrant's behavior. These mediating experiences are what psychiatric epidemiologists refer to as the "stress process," which encompasses the interactions between life-event stresses, intrapsychic and social resources for coping with these stresses, and the manifestation of psychological distress. Detailed accounts of the stress process have been presented elsewhere (e.g., Cervantes and Castro, 1985; Pearlin et al., 1981). Here, it is important to keep in mind a distinction between primary strains, which are so persistent and enveloping as to create enduring problems, and discrete life-event stresses, which persist over a circumscribed period of time (for example, several months to a year) and which are proximate to the individual (Paykel et al., 1969).

A variety of models of the stress process have been proposed in recent years in different contexts. The complexity of such models varies as well, as researchers have multiplied the list of internal and external mechanisms in the creation of stress, and in the cognitive appraisal, psychological and social mediation of the magnitude of stress by the individual. For example, Cervantes and Castro (1985) provide a model of stress and coping related to Mexican American mental health. Their review of the literature repeatedly points to the limited dimensionality of investigations of the stress process, and they propose a multivariate conception. The model begins with the onset of potential stressors (e.g., divorce, unemployment), the intensities of which are subject to cognitive appraisal. Thus, the same source of stress may be judged relatively stressful by one individual or by one cultural group but not another. Internal and external mediators (e.g., personality and family support networks) further shape the imprint that stress leaves on the individual. Mechanisms attempting to cope with stress become activated, the particular style of coping being in many instances culturally prescribed. Depending on the dynamics of these interactions, within and outside the individual, both short-term and long-term effects of stress are felt and perhaps manifested in the form of psychological symptoms. The model is comprehensive, encompassing a multiplicity of internal and external factors leading to distress, and provides reciprocal feedback loops among the major components of the process.

A much simpler model, specifically tied to the stress process involving migration-induced primary strains, was first proposed by Rogler et al. (1983) and subsequently further developed (Rogler et al., 1987). Figure 2.1 presents their model with some adaptations. The stress process, indicated by the elements within the dotted box, is integrated with the migration process. The direct path from migration to psychiatric distress constitutes our second research problem. Within the stress process, the path of intervening experiences to psychological distress constitutes our third research problem. Finally, the indirect path of migration through intervening experiences to psychological distress represents the integration of the second and third research problems, as intervening experiences mitigate the effects of the migration experience on psychological distress. Our discussion of the stress process concentrates on this model, first, because it deals with the migration experience and, second, because it is less formal and more generic, subsuming the components of more complex models. Presented with a minimum of clutter, the model represents the major categories of variables presumed to constitute the stress process. The value of the model is in highlighting issues and processes in need of research, rather than in the enumeration of networks of relationships between the many possible facets of each broad class of variables. Our discussion focuses on the intervening experiences as related to the three primary strains, and concludes with some final observations about research on psychological distress.

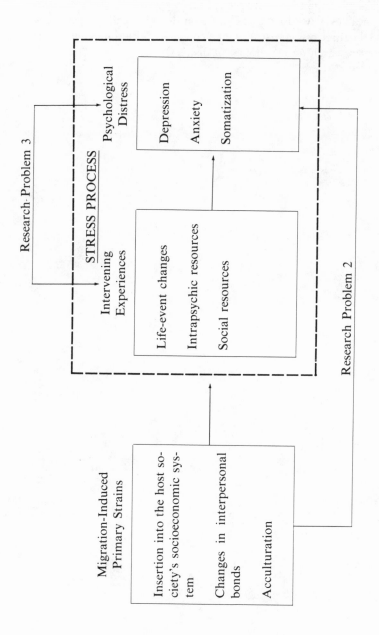

FIG. 2.1   Migration and the stress process.

Significant changes in life events, such as divorce or loss of employment, have been classified in many ways: according to the adaptive requirements of the event; desirability, controllability, and expectedness of the event; and whether the event represents a loss or gain of interpersonal relationships. Despite a number of methodological problems with the literature on life events—distortions in recall of events, causal sequencing of events and psychological symptoms, and tautologous dependencies between operational definitions of events and distress, to name a few—there is a modest legacy of research demonstrating that the significance of recent life events is linked to anxiety (Lauer, 1973), depression (Paykel et al., 1969), schizophrenia (Brown and Birley, 1968; Rogler and Hollingshead, 1985), psychiatric hospitalization (Fontana et al., 1972), psychological impairment (Myers et al., 1971), and psychological distress (Kuo and Tsai, 1986). This research draws our attention to discrete life events as critical components of the stress process.

A major question which arises in this context is: Are the primary strains induced by migration linked to stressful life-event changes? Some of the literature already discussed on the topic of migration and mental health suggests an affirmative answer to this question. For example, considering the first primary strain, if an immigrant is inserted into the bottom of the host society's socioeconomic system, there is a greater likelihood of experiencing a wide range of stressful life events, such as unemployment, downward mobility, necessity of public assistance, and sheer economic survival. Cervantes and Castro (1985) cite literature suggesting that prolonged unemployment, low education, low income, and prejudice and discrimination in the work force increase the risk of psychological disorder precisely because they are stressful events. The collective stress created by such socioeconomic conditions magnifies the risk of psychological disorder, and imposes barriers to effective adaptation to the host society, when the conditions are persistent and chronic. Considering another primary strain, Berry (1980) suggests that "acculturation stress" arises when immigrants must undergo "shifts" in functioning in the effort to adapt to the new language, cognitive styles, personality expectations, identity, and attitudes of the dominant culture. Moreover, Berry links acculturative stress directly to ensuing psychopathological behaviors. Cervantes and Castro cite studies of Mexican Americans and other culturally marginated groups which produced findings consistent with Berry's conclusions. However, we know of no study which assesses the collective impact of all three primary strains on the occurrence of stressful life events. When such studies are conducted, and we hope they will be, they should seek to identify the mechanisms intervening between primary strains and stressful life events in relation to the emergence of psychological distress.

In addition to life-event changes that are stress-provoking, the model of the stress process includes mediating factors consisting of the person's intrapsychic and social resources for interpreting and coping with change. The operation of such mediating factors can be inferred initially from the finding that mere intensity of external stress does a less than satisfactory job of predicting psychological disorder (Pearlin et al., 1981), so it would appear that individuals differ in their reaction to the same external pressures. Cervantes and Castro (1985) note some apparent differences in the appraisal of the significance of stress across cultures. For example, whites tend to appraise life events involving disruption of the nuclear family (e.g., divorce or death) as most stressful, while Mexican Americans accord greater significance to events involving geographic and socioeconomic changes. Another internal mediator of stress, quite independent of one's appraisal of the significance of stress, is that some persons are hardier than others in their confrontations with stressful life events. In research on Asian immigrants to the United States, Kuo and Tsai (1986) conceive of hardy persons as being in control of their lives, as committed to life activities, and as possessing the capacity to welcome change as an exciting challenge. Pearlin et al. (1981) have proposed that such modes of coping with stress by a cultural group are learned from the normative teachings extended by primary group membership. Thus, culturally prescribed modes of coping with stress serve to modify the situation giving rise to stress, to alter the meaning of problems (appraisal) in the interest of reducing stress, and to facilitate the management of socially acceptable expressions of stress-promoted symptoms.

Personality traits, as shaped by the culture, also have been implicated as mediators of the effects of stress on psychological disorder. In their review of personality trait and assessment research on Mexican Americans, Cervantes and Castro (1985) summarize studies focusing on how Mexican Americans differ from whites in certain personality characteristics, such as locus of control, achievement motivation, cognitive style, fatalism, conformity, and field dependence/independence. However, they caution against stereotypic generalizations and attempts to define the "Mexican personality." Similar characterizations have been proposed about Puerto Ricans and Cubans in the interest of sensitizing non-Hispanic clinicians to the nuances common to Hispanic cultures, but caveats must be interjected to avoid unappropriate stereotypy if such generalizations are made indiscriminately (Malgady et al., 1987). Although the literature is replete with studies proposing specific personality dimensions on which Hispanics differ in general from the majority culture, there appears to be little or no discussion of how such differences in personality structure—if indeed they are not measurement artifacts—mediate the effects of stress on psychological disorder. If it is true that Mexican Americans, for example, generally are fatalistic, externally oriented, and overcompliant, how does this personality profile exacerbate or buffer the potentially debilitating effect of stressful life events on the individual? Given that the literature on comparative personality differences between ethnic populations is controversial and prone to stereotyping, as well as the questionable validity of personality assessments of Hispanics (Cervantes and Castro, 1985; Olmedo, 1981; Malgady et al., 1987), the answer to this question is likely to remain elusive until more fundamental questions are resolved.

Without doubting the importance of psychological resources in mediating the relationship between primary strains, life events, and psychological disorder, the mediator most commonly examined in the research literature and more easily measured than covert psychological processes is the social support network surrounding the individual. With respect to the family network, we have already asserted that migration results in the disruption of primary bonds—the separation of close relatives, postponement of marriage, and delay of family formation. After migration the time required to reassemble such basic intrafamilial bonds is likely to vary considerably according to an array of considerations associated with the resettlement process in the host society. The family is perhaps the most salient source of identity and social support for many Hispanics, but strong familism not only reduces stress but paradoxically also may inhibit a person's interactions with social-support networks outside the family, such as traditional mental health service agencies (Cervantes and Castro, 1985).

In relation to the acculturation process, Griffith and Villavicencio (1985) reported that as acculturation increases, especially among second- and third-generation Hispanics, the extended family network increases in scope. But despite these seemingly greater resources for social support in coping with stress, highly acculturated Hispanics are less likely to rely on the extended family network for social support. Other sources of social support external to the family are discussed in more detail in the following chapter dealing with Hispanic utilization of mental health services.

What is needed in future research on the stress process are life-span studies of how primary strains resulting from rupturing intimate social and familial bonds evolve to shape the nature of immigrants' supportive networks, including the conditions under which management of stress is either facilitated or impugned. This need is perhaps most pronounced with respect to female-headed households, since many Hispanic families are headed by single women. The seriousness of the problem must be emphasized because, compared to intact Hispanic families, single-headed families are disproportionately poor (Angel and Tienda, 1982), less likely to be in the labor force (Tienda and Glass, 1985), and the female heads of such households present high levels of anxiety (Gurak, 1984). Thus, female heads of household experience even more intense primary strains than those previously discussed because of their extremely low socioeconomic position and, presumably, fewer interpersonal resources for coping with stress. From an epidemiological perspective, we need to learn more about the role of the migration experience and settlement process in encouraging such households to form. Then we need to determine whether the major contributor to mental health problems is the socioeconomic strain, the lack of interpersonal resources, or some combination of these and other factors.

Psychological distress is what most epidemiological studies ultimately attempt to explain. We have already referred to a body of literature on the mental health status characteristics of Hispanic populations, and we have pointed out a number of methodological and substantive limitations of this research. We offer one further observation in the context of the stress process. Two approaches to the study of psychological disorder among Hispanic populations should be distinguished. The first approach, which prevails by far in epidemiological research, begins with preselected measures of mental illness, such as anxiety or depression, and proceeds to test stress-related theoretical formulations. The second approach, which is more fundamental but less ubiquitous, begins with the assumption that our ignorance of the indigenous configuration of mental health problems should temper our preconceived notions about which dimensions of mental health are most salient. If research begins with a commitment to pre-established measures of psychological disorder, such research produces data specific to the preconceptions of the researcher, with no evidence that the data correctly reflect the most salient mental health problems in the Hispanic populations studied. The new cross-cultural psychiatry is giving this issue the immediate and continuing attention it deserves (Kleinman and Good, 1985). The proliferation of findings from the first approach will no doubt create the impression among mental health researchers—especially those only dimly aware of cultural issues—that the objectives of comparative epidemiological research have been met. If we are to explore fully the intricate connections between the migration experience, the stress process, and mental health through programmatic research, data collected by the second approach represent an essential supplement to the customary measures of mental disorder and symptomatology. The influence of primary strains and of intervening experiences upon psychological distress needs to be examined in the broadest possible context which is sensitive to Hispanic mental health problems.

The theoretical formulations pertinent to migration-induced primary strains and the stress process can be combined in focusing upon the question raised at the beginning of this chapter: Does the migration experience create psychological distress? The answer to this question depends upon how the immigrant is situated with respect to the model linking the migration experience to the stress process. An immigrant who is at high risk for the development of psychological distress is one who is inserted into the bottom of the host society's socioeconomic system, has acculturation problems which swing him or her away from an adaptive bicultural identity, and is separated from socially supportive networks by migration. Along with such primary strains, he or she is a person experiencing a high quotient of life-event stresses but is unable to cope effectively with such strains and stresses because of limited intrapsychic and social resources.

Summary

Three research problems at the core of the conceptual framework's first phase—the emergence of psychological distress—were formulated in this chapter: the comparative distribution of mental health problems in Hispanic and other populations; the migration experience and mental health; and the stress process. In the course of formulating the problems, we have progressively brought the findings of epidemiological studies to bear upon issues of Hispanic mental health, identified methodological problems in such studies, and made recommendations pertinent to future research development. The next chapter extends this pattern of presentation into the framework's second phase, the help-seeking efforts prompted by the experience of mental health problems.

References

Aneshensel, C.C. and Frerichs, R.R. (1982). Stress, support, and depression: A longitudinal causal model. *Journal of Community Psychology* 10: 363-376.

Aneshensel, C.C. and Stone, J.D. (1982). Stress and depression: A test of buffering model of social support. *Archives of General Psychiatry* 39: 1392-1396.

Angel, R. and Tienda, M. (1982). Determinants of extended household structure: Cultural pattern or economic need? *American Journal of Sociology* 87: 1360-1383.

Baskin, D., Bluestone, H. and Nelson, M. (1981). Ethnicity and psychiatric diagnosis. *Journal of Clinical Psychology* 37: 529-537.

Bell, R.A., Leroy, J.B. and Stephenson, J.J. (1982). Evaluating the effect of social support upon life events and depressive symptoms. *Journal of Community Psychology* 10: 325-340.

Berry, J.W. (1980). Acculturation as varieties of adaptation. In A.M. Padilla (Ed.), *Acculturation: Theory, Models and Some New Findings* (pp.9-25). Boulder: Westview Press.

Billings, A.G. and Moos, R.H. (1985). Life stressors and social resources affecting posttreatment outcomes among depressed patients. *Journal of Abnormal Psychology* 94: 140-153.

Bromet, E., Schulberg, H.C. and Dunn, L. (1982). Reactions of psychiatric patients to the Three Mile Island nuclear accident. *Archives of General Psychiatry* 39: 725-730.

Brown, G.N. and Birley, J.L. (1968). Crises and life changes and the onset of schizophrenia. *Journal of Health and Social Behavior* 9: 203-214.

Burnam, M.A., Hough, R.L., Karno, M., Escobar, J.I. and Telles, C.A. (1987). Acculturation and lifetime prevalence of psychiatric disorders among Mexican Americans in Los Angeles. *Journal of Health and Social Behavior* 28: 89-102.

Canino, G.J., Bird, H.R., Shrout, P.E., Rubio-Stipec, M., Geil, K.P. and Bravo, M. (1987a). The prevalence of alcohol abuse and/or dependence in Puerto Rico. In M. Gaviria and J.D. Arana (Eds.), *Health and Behavior: Research Agenda for Hispanics* (pp.127-144). Chicago: Simon Bolivar Research Monograph (No. 1), University of Illinois at Chicago.

Canino, G.J., Bird, H.R., Shrout, P.E. Rubio-Stipec, M., Bravo, M., Martinez, R., Sesman, M., Guzman, A., Guevara, L.J. and Costas, H. (1987b). The Spanish Diagnostic Interview Schedule: Reliability and concordance with clinical diagnoses in Puerto Rico. *Archives of General Psychiatry* 44: 720-726.

Canino, G.J., Bird, H.R., Shrout, P.E. Rubio-Stipec, M., Bravo, M., Martinez, R., Sesman, M. and Guevara, L.J. (1987c). The prevalence of specific psychiatric disorders in Puerto Rico. *Archives of General Psychiatry* 44: 727-735.

Catalano, R. and Dooley, D. (1977). Economic predictors of depressed mood and stressful life events in a metropolitan community. *Journal of Health and Social Behavior* 18: 292-307.

Cervantes, R.C. and Castro, F.G. (1985). Stress, coping, and Mexican American mental health: A systematic review. *Hispanic Journal of Behavioral Sciences* 2: 199-217.

Cuellar, I., Harris, L. and Jasso, R. (1980). An acculturation scale for Mexican American normal and clinical populations. *Hispanic Journal of Behavioral Sciences* 2: 199-217.

Dohrenwend, B.P. (1966). Social status and psychological disorder: An issue of substance and an issue of method. *American Sociological Review* 31: 14-34.

Dohrenwend, B.P. and Dohrenwend, B.S. (1969). *Social Status and Psychological Disorder: A Causal Inquiry.* New York: John Wiley.

Dohrenwend, B.P., Dohrenwend, B.S., Gould, M.S., Link, B., Neugebauer, R. and Wunsch-Hitzig, R. (1980). *Mental Illness in the United States.* New York: Praeger.

Dooley, D. and Catalano, R. (1980). Economic change as a cause of behavioral disorder. *Psychological Bulletin* 87: 450-468.

Durkheim, E. (1951). *Suicide: A Study in Sociology.* (Translated by J.A. Spaulding and G. Simpson.) New York: The Free Press.

Eaton, W.W. and Kessler, L.G. (Eds.) (1985). *Epidemiologic Field Methods in Psychiatry.* New York: Academic Press.

Fontana, A.F., Marcus, J.L., Noel, B. and Rakusin, J.M. (1972). Prehospitalization coping styles of psychiatric patients: The goal-directedness of life events. *Journal of Nervous and Mental Diseases* 155: 311-321.

Fried, M. (1980). Stress, strain, and role adaptation: Conceptual issues. In G.V. Coelho and P.I. Ahmed (Eds.), *Uprooting and Development* (pp. 67-96). New York: Plenum Press.

Griffith, J. and Villavicencio, S. (1985). Relationship among acculturation, sociodemographic characteristics and social supports in Mexican American adults. *Hispanic Journal of Behavioral Sciences* 7: 75-92.

Gross, H., Knatterud, G. and Donner, L. (1969). The effect of race and sex on the variation of diagnosis and disposition in a psychiatric emergency room. *Journal of Nervous and Mental Diseases* 148: 638-642.

Gurak, D.T. (1984). Acculturation and mental health among Dominican and Colombian immigrants in New York City. Paper presented at the meeting of the American Sociological Association, San Antonio, August.

Gurak, D.T. and Kritz, M.M. (1984). Kinship networks and the settlement process: Dominican and Colombian immigrants in New York City. *Research Bulletin* 7: 7-11 (Hispanic Research Center, Fordham University, Bronx, N.Y.).

Haberman, P. (1976). Psychiatric symptoms among Puerto Ricans in Puerto Rico and New York City. *Ethnicity* 3: 133-144.

Hollingshead, A.B. and Redlich, F.C. (1958). *Social Class and Mental Illness.* New York: John Wiley.

Jaco, E.G. (1960). *The Social Epidemiology of Mental Disorders.* New York: Russell Sage Foundation.

Karno, M., Burnam, M.A., Hough, R.L., Escobar, J.I. and Golding, J.M. (1987). Mental disorder among Mexican Americans and non-Hispanic whites in Los Angeles. In M. Gaviria and J.D. Arana (Eds.), *Health and Behavior: Research Agenda for Hispanics,* (pp. 110-126). Simon Bolivar Research Monograph No. 1, University of Illinois at Chicago.

Kessler, R.C. (1979). Stress, social status, and psychological distress. *Journal of Health and Social Behavior* 20: 259-272.

Kessler, R.C. and Cleary, P.D. (1980). Social class and psychological stress. *American Sociological Review* 45: 463-478.

Kleiner, R. and Parker, S. (1959). Migration and mental illness: A new look. *American Sociological Review* 24: 687-690.

Kleiner, R. and Parker, S. (1965). Goal striving and psychosomatic symptoms in migrant and non-migrant populations. In M. Kantor (Ed.), *Mobility and Mental Health* (pp. 78-85). Springfield, Illinois: Charles C. Thomas.

Kleinman, A. and Good, B. (Eds.) (1985). *Culture and Depression.* Berkeley: University of California Press.

Kuo, W.H. and Tsai, Y. (1986). Social networking, hardiness, and immigrant's mental health. *Journal of Health and Social Behavior* 27: 133-149.

Lauer, R.H. (1973). The social readjustment scale and anxiety: A cross-cultural study. *Journal of Psychosomatic Research* 17: 171-174.

Lee, E. (1963). Socioeconomic and migration differentials in mental disease, New York State, 1949-61. *Milbank Memorial Fund Quarterly* 41: 249-268.

Malgady, R.G., Rogler, L.H. and Costantino, G. (1987). Ethnocultural and linguistic bias in mental health evaluation of Hispanics. *American Psychologist* 42: 228-234.

Malzberg, B. (1962). The mental health of the Negro: A study of first admissions to hospitals for mental disease in New York State, 1949-51. Albany, N.Y.: Research Foundation for Mental Hygiene.

Marin, G., Sabogal, F., Marin V.B., Otero-Sabogal, R. and Perez-Stable, E.J. (1987). Development of a short acculturation scale for Hispanics. *Hispanic Journal of Behavioral Sciences* 9: 183-205.

Moscicki, E.K., Rae, D., Regier, D.A. and Locke, B.Z. (1987). The Hispanic Health and Nutrition Examination Survey: Depression among Mexican Americans, Cuban Americans, Puerto Ricans. In M. Gaviria and J.D. Arana (Eds.), *Health and Behavior: Research Agenda for Hispanics* (pp. 145-159). University of Illinois at Chicago (Simon Bolivar Research Monograph No. 1).

Murphy, H.B. (1973). Migration and major mental disorders: A reappraisal. In C. Zwingmann and M. Pfister-Ammende (Eds.), *Uprooting and After* (pp. 204-220). New York: Springer-Verlag.

Myers, J.K., Lindenthal, J.J. and Pepper, M.P. (1971). Life events and psychiatric impairment. *Journal of Nervous and Mental Diseases* 152: 149-157.

Odegaard, O. (1932). Emigration and insanity: A study of mental disease among the Norwegian-born population in Minnesota. *Acta Psychiatrica et Neurologica, Scandanavia* (Suppl.) 4: 1-206.

Olmedo, E.L. (1981). Testing linguistic minorities. *American Psychologist* 36: 1078-1085.

Ortiz, V. and Arce, C.J. (1984). Language orientation and mental health status among persons of Mexican descent. *Hispanic Journal of Behavioral Sciences* 6: 127-143.

Padilla, A.M. (1980). The role of cultural awareness and ethnic loyalty in acculturation. In A.M. Padilla (Ed.), *Acculturation: Theory, Models and Some New Findings* (pp. 47-84). Boulder, Colorado: Westview Press.

Parker, S., Kleiner, R. and Needelman, B. (1969). Migration and mental illness: Some reconsiderations and suggestions for further analysis. *Social Science and Medicine* 3: 1-9.

Paykel, E.S., Myers, J.K., Dienelt, M.N., Klerman, G.L. and Lindenthal, J.J. (1969). Life events depression: A controlled study. *Archives of General Psychiatry* 21: 753-760.

Pearlin, L.I., Lieberman, M.A., Menaghan, E.G. and Mullan, J.T. (1981). The stress process. *Journal of Health and Social Behavior* 22: 337-356.

Reubens, P. (1980). Psychological needs of the new immigrants. *Migration Today* 8: 8-14.

Roberts, R. (1980). Prevalence of psychological distress among Mexican Americans. *Journal of Health and Social Behavior* 21: 134-145.

Roberts, R. (1987). An epidemiological perspective on the mental health of people of Mexican origin. In R. Rodriguez and M.T. Coleman (Eds.), *Mental Health Issues of the Mexican Origin Population in Texas.* Austin: Hogg Foundation for Mental Health.

Rogg, E.M. and Cooney, R.S. (1980). *Adaptation and Adjustment of Cubans: West New York, New Jersey.* Bronx, N.Y.: Hispanic Research Center, Fordham University (Monograph No. 5).

Rogler, L.H. (1984). *Migrant in the City,* 2nd ed. Maplewood, N.J.: Waterfront Press.

Rogler, L.H. and Cooney, R.S. (1984). *Puerto Rican Families in New York City: Intergenerational Processes.* Maplewood, N.J.: Waterfront Press (Hispanic Research Center Monograph No. 11).

Rogler, L.H., Cooney, R.S., Costantino, G., Earley B., Gurak, D., Malgady, R.G. and Rodriguez, O. (1983). *A Conceptual Framework for Mental Health Research on Hispanic Populations.* Bronx, N.Y.: Hispanic Research Center, Fordham University (Monograph No. 10).

Rogler, L.H. and Hollingshead, A.B. (1985). *Trapped: Puerto Rican Families and Schizophrenia,* 3rd ed. Maplewood, New Jersey: Waterfront Press.

Rogler, L.H., Gurak, D.T. and Cooney, R.S. (1987). The migration experience and mental health: Formulations relevant to Hispanics and other immigrants. In M. Gaviria and J.D. Arana (Eds.), *Health and Behavior: Research Agenda for Hispanics* (pp. 72-84). Simon Bolivar Research Monograph (No. 1), University of Illinois at Chicago.

Sanua, V. (1970). Immigration, migration, and mental illness: A review of the literature with special emphasis on schizophrenia. In E. Brody (Ed.), *Behavior in New Environments: Adaptation of Migrant Populations* (2nd ed.) (pp. 291-352). Beverly Hills: Sage Publications.

Schwab, J.J. and Schwab, M.E. (1978). *Sociocultural Roots of Mental Illness.* New York: Plenum Publishing Corp.

Srole, L., Langner, T., Michael, S., Opler, M. and Rennic, T. (1962). *Mental Health in the Metropolis: The Midtown Manhattan Study.* New York: McGraw-Hill.

Szapocznik, J., Kurtines, W.M. and Fernandez, T. (1980). Bicultural involvement in Hispanic American youths. *International Journal of Intercultural Relations* 4: 353-365.

Szapocznik, J., Scopetta, M.A., Kurtines, W. and Aranalde, M.A. (1978). Theory and measurement of acculturation. *Interamerican Journal of Psychology* 12: 113-130.

Tienda, M. and Glass, J. (1985). Household structure and labor force participation of black, Hispanic, and white mothers. *Demography* 22: 381-394.

Torres-Matrullo, C.M. (1976). Acculturation and psychopathology among Puerto Rican women in mainland United States. *American Journal of Orthopsychiatry* 46: 710-719.

Vega, W., Warheit, G.J., Auth, J.B. and Meinhardt, K. (1984). The prevalence of depressive symptoms among Mexican Americans and Anglos. *American Journal of Epidemiology* 120: 592-607.

Vega, W., Warheit, G.J. and Palacio, R. (1985). Psychiatric symptomatology among Mexican American farm workers. *Social Science and Medicine* 20: 39-45.

Verdonk, A. (1979). Migration and mental illness. *International Journal of Social Psychiatry* 25: 295-305.

Warheit, G.J., Vega, W., Auth, J.B. and Meinhardt, K. (1985). Psychiatric symptoms and dysfunctions among Anglos and Mexican Americans: An epidemiological study. In J.R. Greenley (Ed.), *Research in Community and Mental Health* (pp. 3-32). Greenwich, Connecticut: JAI Press.

Chapter 3

Phase Two: Help-Seeking Behavior

Sixteen days after the birth of her first child, Mrs. Beatriz Lopez suddenly felt a "great despair rushing into my head" and a fear that her baby was going to be harmed. She wept uncontrollably. Her sister in-law explained that the blood which had accumulated during childbirth had flowed to her head, but that gradually the blood would drain to other parts of her body and she would be well again. This did not occur. The despair continued, along with anxiety, depression, suicidal wishes, and incessant weeping. Mrs. Lopez was married to an alcoholic husband who repeatedly beat her, once causing her to miscarry when seven months pregnant and another time, cracking her skull. Attempted reconciliations following upon marital disruptions did not work. Once, having abandoned her to return to Puerto Rico, he persuaded her to return to the island to live in a "beautiful home" he had rented. The home turned out to be a shack in the middle of a cemetery.

Eleven years after the birth of her first child and the first psychiatric episode, the physician attending to the birth of her fourth child advised her to see a psychiatrist, which she did for six months. Thirteen years after this, Mrs. Lopez began therapy in a community mental health center. During twenty-four years she had contact with a mental health professional only once. During this time, she received help and social support from her mother, brothers, and children. Her eldest son took her to a spiritualist for help but it did not work because "spiritualists at one time were genuinely concerned with helping people, but now they want to get paid." She was active in her church group, and worried deeply about her children's problems which involved drug addiction, infidelity, and violence. She endured her emotional problems as part of what life brings. Recently she went to a non-Hispanic therapist, but the therapist reprimanded her. Now she is going to a Hispanic therapist who is very understanding. For the first time in many years, she can now talk about her problems without weeping.

* * *

The second phase of our hypothetical temporal sequence focuses on the

45

experience of mental health problems and the help-seeking efforts initiated to alleviate the distress caused by such problems. The research literature suggests that when Hispanics experience psychological problems, they are less likely than other ethnic group individuals to seek the help of professional mental health service providers. Thus, the first research problem posed in this phase focuses on Hispanic utilization of mental health facilities and the second, upon factors which explain such utilization.

We begin the examination of the first research problem by considering the evidence regarding Hispanic utilization of mental health facilities. Most studies which show that Hispanics underutilize mental health facilities base their claim on findings that Hispanics have lower rates of admissions to facilities than other ethnic groups. Few studies, however, address the question of whether Hispanics have low admission rates in relation to high rates of mental illness—which would indicate service underutilization—or whether Hispanics have low admission rates in comparison to low rates of mental illness—which would not indicate underutilization. This research question recalls the first question posed in Chapter 2: What is the extent of mental health problems among Hispanics? In relation to the underutilization issue, however, the question has to be put in a broader context: When admission rates are considered in relation to prevalence rates, to what extent is underutilization a problem for Hispanics?

The second research problem relevant to Phase Two stems from different opinions about which factors best explain Hispanic underutilization rates. The research problem can be stated in the context of the two major explanations of Hispanic underutilization of mental health facilities: alternative resource theory and barrier theory. The theory of alternative resources explains underutilization in terms of the indigenous Hispanic social organizations—or primary group structures—that serve as therapeutic alternatives to the official mental health agency system. The argument is that Hispanics with psychological problems first turn to proximate and culturally familiar indigenous organizations, i.e., family, friends, religious and spiritualist groups, and, if there is no satisfactory solution to the problem, then, they turn to mental health facilities. Barrier theory, on the other hand, views underutilization as the result of two types of obstacles to professional mental health care: certain Hispanic cultural values and beliefs which predispose Hispanics not to seek professional care and institutional characteristics of the service delivery system which impede utilization by Hispanics.

The explanations are not mutually exclusive. Each differs in the class of variables it considers to be relevant. We shall see that research findings question some of the assumptions upon which alternative resource and barrier theories are based and point to interrelationships among the factors emphasized by each theory. Thus, the second research problem in Phase Two focuses on how to integrate these theories into a comprehensive and dynamic explanation of Hispanic underutilization.

The Evidence of Hispanic Underutilization

Studies examining Hispanic utilization of mental health facilities generally have concluded that Hispanics underutilize mental health services in comparison to most other ethnic groups. Since the studies reach their conclusions on the basis of divergent definitions of underutilization, it is useful to enumerate the different ways utilization has been measured. Some studies compare Hispanic admission rates, based upon the proportion of Hispanic users of a particular mental health facility or a number of such facilities, with the Hispanics' proportionate size in the population at large or the relevant catchment area. When the first proportion is smaller than the second proportion, the group is said to underutilize; when the first proportion is larger than the second, it is said to overutilize. Admission rates have also been used to make intergroup (ethnic or racial) comparisons in determining over- and underutilization. Some studies arrive at more refined estimates by comparing ethnic groups with respect to the number of admissions per 100,000 of their respective subpopulations. Other studies do not make reference to the underlying population bases, but only compare the percentage of each ethnic group admitted to one or a number of facilities.

These measures are synonymous with the rates-under-treatment measures cited in Chapter 2. Just as rates under treatment are inadequate indicators of the true prevalence of mental illness, they are inadequate measures of over- or underutilization. The key datum missing in both types of measures is the prevalence of mental health problems in the relevant population groups. This shortcoming should be kept in mind as we review the evidence of Hispanic underutilization.

Among studies using national data on Hispanic utilization, Bachrach's (1975) concluded that Hispanics were underrepresented in their admissions to inpatient psychiatric units of state and county hospitals throughout the United States. Since that time, several national surveys have been conducted by the National Institute of Mental Health with the results generally agreeing with those of Bachrach. Hispanics were found to underutilize outpatient psychiatric services, private psychiatric hospitals, and the psychiatric services of non-public, non-federal general hospitals (NIMH, 1980). At the same time, Hispanics were found to overutilize the inpatient psychiatric services of public, non-federal general hospitals. This would suggest that they have more severe problems requiring hospitalization.

Most of our knowledge about Hispanic utilization rates comes from studies of the Mexican American population. Lopez (1981) reviewed 49 studies, 28 of which reported underutilization of facilities as indicated by comparing the facility or catchment area admission rates of Mexican Americans with those of Anglos and other ethnic groups, or by comparing the proportion of Mexican Americans in the facilities with their proportion in the corresponding catchment area population. Utilization rates proportionate to Mexican American representation were more likely in southwestern states or in single facilities, and underutilization was more likely in Los Angeles and other California communities. For example, one of the studies cited by Lopez showed that in 1977 Mexican Americans represented 22 percent of Los Angeles County's population, but only 13 percent of outpatient clinic admission and 7 percent of inpatient facility admissions.

Fewer studies of Puerto Rican utilization are available. The early studies of New York City's Puerto Rican population found them to have higher rates of reported psychiatric admissions than other ethnic groups in the city, but more recent studies show underutilization by Puerto Ricans and other Hispanic groups in New York City. Among the early studies, Fitzpatrick and Gould (1968) analyzed the first admissions of New York City children to NY State psychiatric hospitals in 1967 and concluded that the admissions rate was considerably higher for Spanish-speaking children than for the non-Spanish-speaking. Two studies using administratively collected data in specific New York City catchment areas (NIMH, 1976 a,b) also found that the admission rates for non-Hispanic whites were considerably lower than those for blacks and Puerto Ricans. Alers (1978), using New York City figures for admissions to all local community mental health and retardation facilities, reported that the admission rate for Puerto Ricans was approximately twice the rate for non-Hispanics.

More recent admission rates published by New York State and based on more comprehensive data collection clearly indicate that Puerto Ricans and other Hispanic groups in New York City underutilize mental health services. The one-week survey of patient characteristics conducted by New York State's Office of Mental Health estimated that in 1981, 861 out of every 100,000 Hispanics were admitted to outpatient clinics, while the admission rates for blacks, whites, and Native and Asian Americans were 1104, 1046, and 303 per 100,000, respectively (NYSOMH, 1982). Admission rates for inpatient facilities showed even greater ethnic differentials, with 170 admissions for every 100,000 Hispanics, and 324, 231, and 70 admissions for every 100,000 blacks, whites, and Native and Asian Americans, respectively. The New York State data thus provide evidence that, with the exception of Native and Asian Americans, Hispanics have the lowest utilization rates relative to population size.

Although the most current utilization research concludes that in general Hispanics underutilize mental health services, more incisive research questions should be asked in order to resolve the discrepancies among study findings. For example, does the difference in utilization among catchment areas reflect differences in prevalence rates? Or are the barriers to utilization more formidable in some areas than others? Or are there differences in indigenous social organizations which are creating such differences? We can raise these questions, but we cannot answer them. Thus, Hispanic groups in specific areas, characterized as overutilizers, because of their proportionately higher admissions, may be underutilizers relative to their mental health needs. Admission rates, therefore, must be seen in relation to the issues raised in Phase One regarding true prevalence rates in specific groups. Conclusions relevant to over- and underutilization would then be premised upon the magnitude of differences between the two rates, with admission rates expected to be consistently lower than prevalence rates. Research to provide data for the computation of such rates is needed if we are to arrive at sound policy decisions regarding Hispanic utilization of mental health services. Although the studies point to a problem of Hispanic underutilization, none has examined the problem with adequate measures of both mental illness and admission rates.

We now turn to the question of the second research problem focusing on the two explanations for underutilization: alternative resource theory and barrier theory.

Alternative Resource and Barrier Theories

To view the problem of underutilization from the perspective of alternative resources is to view it in the context of informal, crescive social organizations, as opposed to formally constituted bureaucratic service structures. The psychologically afflicted person's help-seeking efforts are seen in the context of interpersonal relations and networks—the family, the circle of friends, neighbors and acquaintances, the coparent system, the indigenous folk healing institutions—all in juxtaposition with the mental health agency system. The broadest question to be posed, consequently, is how does the interrelationship among these primary groups or social organizations affect the person's help-seeking efforts. Is getting help from the family likely to decrease the probability of the afflicted person's seeking help from friends or folk healers or the mental health agency system? Do such social groupings represent alternative sources of help or are they conjoined in the provision of help? In comparison to other groups, to what extent do Hispanics use such social groupings? Does the pattern of use from one resource to another differ across ethnic groups and social classes? The literature on these questions is confusing, but its size nonetheless attests to the importance ascribed to social organization—and, hence, to alternative resource theory—in understanding patterns of mental health utilization.

The family is the foremost social organization in Hispanic culture seen as relevant to underutilization. The prevailing view is well presented by Hoppe and Heller (1975):

> Familism is a positive form of social organization that facilitates their (Hispanics') adaptation to the conditions of marginal (objectively alienated) existence and its subjectively alienating consequences. Family ties serve supportive and protective functions against the risk of failure, economic loss, embarrassment, and vulnerability to criticism encountered in the broader society. Such ties serve as a "buffer" between the objectively alienated Mexican American and the Anglo middle-class society. (p.306)

It is understandable why the family, in the context of alternative resource theory, is viewed almost exclusively as a supportive, help-giving system, since the giving and receiving of help is an integral component of familial bonds (Rogler and Hollingshead, 1985). But the generalizing of this view to encompass all issues relevant to mental health creates idealistic stereotypes which are scientifically counterproductive and cloud the possibility of studying the family as a source of mental distress. Not all that goes on in Hispanic families is supportive, harmonious, and consensually based. As in other groups, there are also conflict and dissension, bitter recrimination, and violence—a view which is consistent, for example, with the rapid increase of single-parent households among New York City's Puerto Ricans (Mann and Salvo, 1985). The increasing problems besetting the Puerto Rican family are also suggested by the rising number of divorces in relation to marriages among New York City Puerto Ricans: in 1960 there was one person divorced for every 24 persons married; in 1970, one person divorced for every 15 persons married; and in 1980, one person divorced for every 12 persons married (U.S. Bureau of the Census, 1963, 1973, 1980).

To some researchers, the major difference between Anglos and Mexican

Americans in help-seeking behavior is to be found in the latter group's seeking of help primarily from the family rather than from friends (Keefe et al., 1978; Keefe, 1978). However, conclusions on this point differ. For example, Padilla et al. (1976) state that to deal with emotional problems, Mexican Americans depend upon physicians, relatives, friends, and religious practitioners for treatment. In contrast, Keefe et al. (1978) assert that the Mexican Americans' main resource is their extended kin network; and that little support is derived from other informal sources. Although the importance of the family is reaffirmed, the importance of friends or informal sources as help-givers remains inconclusive.

Much of the literature on the family in Puerto Rico parallels findings on Mexican Americans. Rogler and Hollingshead (1985) documented how families living in the most impoverished neighborhoods and public housing developments in San Juan, Puerto Rico, enmesh their members in a system of help-giving exchanges. The system incorporates the nuclear family into the extended family, because mutual help criss-crosses blood and affinal relationships. Mutual help, in fact, has the force of a sacred obligatory norm: it is sustained by the double edge of guilt and gratitude. That is, not to help a relative in need evokes feelings of guilt; in turn, to be helped by a relative induces feelings of gratitude. The norm applies through time because the person is bound permanently to his or her family of origin; and it applies through space, because relatives who are separated by geographical distance behave in accordance with the norm. The norm's impact is evident in the finding that at the time the study's data were collected, 88 percent of the nuclear families were either giving or receiving material goods in contact with their relatives. The type of help given is linked to sex roles in the family: the women provide family-centered, socioemotional support; the men, the type of help associated with their instrumental roles of linking the family to institutions outside the family.

The findings are not unique. Many studies have documented the family's essential role in the institutional character of Puerto Rican society. The family is central to the island's stratification system, social mobility patterns, and the transition from an agrarian to an industrial society (Tumin and Feldman, 1961); it is the main context of economic consumption (Roberts and Stefani, 1949) and socialization of the young (Wolf, 1952); it binds together reciprocal patterns of help in facilitating rural-to-urban migration and adaptation (Rogler and Hollingshead, 1985); it extends itself into the ritual coparent system of *compadrazgo* to enlarge the scope of its social security function (Mintz, 1956); it is the object of devotion in an overarching system of cultural values (Brameld, 1959); it is the primary setting for the care of the mentally ill (Rogler and Hollingshead, 1985); and it shapes the character of entrepreneurial activities through its system of paternalistic relationships (Cochran, 1959). Despite rapid social change, Puerto Rican society at the root level still centers upon the family and its functions.

Very little is known about the Puerto Rican family in New York City (Rogler, 1978), particularly about its vitality as a help-giving system; how geographical and social mobility affects the system; and how it changes, if at all, from the first to the second generation which now comprises about half of the Puerto Rican population in the city. Most speculations, supported by patches of data, favor the view that migration and acculturation are altering the extended family system (Fitzpatrick, 1971). Rogler and Cooney (1984) have attempted to analyze how intergenerational changes in acculturation among 100 intergenerationally linked New York Puerto Rican nuclear families influenced help-giving patterns. The study found a higher level of help-giving among the Puerto Rican families than among Anglo families in another study using the same instruments.

However, some studies suggest that the influence of the Hispanic family on help-seeking is not a simple process. For example, Keefe (1979) found no statistically significant relationship between mental health clinic contacts and indicators of Mexican American extended family characteristics such as the number of relatives living nearby, the number of kin visits, and the number of instances of family aid. Examining the use of another type of service, health care, Hoppe and Heller (1975) found that frequency of family visits among Mexican Americans was associated with the use of prenatal health care, but was negatively related to consulting a physician when ill. They suggest no explanation for the contradictory influences of the extended family on the two health behaviors. Rodriguez (1987) found that among Hispanics in an inner-city area, extended family activities and supports from neighbors and friends were negatively related to use of mental health services only among those with few or no mental health symptoms. Among those with a high number of symptoms, family and friend network activities were associated with use of services, suggesting that Hispanics' social networks complement professional care by acting as referral information and advice sources. His findings thus modify the original formulation of alternative resource theory by specifying the conditions under which Hispanic social networks provide alternatives to professional care.

Another supportive network commonly cited as important in traditional Hispanic culture is the *compadrazgo* or coparent system. Along with material, moral, and spiritual responsibilities of the godparents toward the godchild, functioning as a form of indigenous social security, the coparent system binds the godparents and the godchild's parents into a pattern of mutual respect and help. Fitzpatrick (1971) states that Puerto Ricans in this system "constitute a network of ritual kinship, as serious and important as that of natural kinship around a person or a group" (pp.81-82). As a traditional idealized system, the statement is true. However, Rogler and Hollingshead's (1985) previously cited study conducted in Puerto Rico found little evidence of a viable, help-giving coparent system; similarly, Rogler and Cooney (1984), focusing upon New York City's Puerto Ricans, showed little involvement by coparents in help-giving exchanges. The same appears to be the case among Mexican Americans (Keefe et al., 1978). Unless new and more convincing evidence is produced by research, the coparent system among Puerto Ricans and Mexican Americans can more appropriately be viewed as having essentially ceremonial meaning, a ritualized cultural form defining respectful formal relationships between the relevant parties.

Perhaps the most disputed area in the theory of alternative resources is the role of spiritualist and folk healer. The subject has received a remarkable amount of attention ever since the Rogler and Hollingshead (1985) study first documented empirically the psychotherapeutic functions of spiritualist sessions in relation to the problems of the mentally ill. The study demonstrated that among persons at the bottom of the San Juan stratification heap, the institution of spiritualism is the most prevalent form of social organization outside the family which helps persons experiencing emotional stress and mental illness (Rogler and Hollingshead, 1960, 1961, 1985). As an ideology, spiritualism assumes an invisible world of good and bad spirits who intrude into human affairs and can be employed by mediums who have developed psychic faculties to cure illness, arbitrate personal disputes, and explain events incongruous with common sense. As an institution, spiritualism is directly interwoven into the trials and tribulations of persons in the San Juan slums and public housing projects; the medium provides spiritualistic interpretations which are simple, credible, and given in a setting free of the stigma associated with psychiatric treatment at hospitals or clinics. In Puerto Rico, persons of modest means almost invariably turned to spiritualism before contacting a psychiatrist or mental health worker. It is not known whether the urbanization process has eroded the pervasive use of spiritualism in Puerto Rico. Descriptive accounts of Puerto Rican life in New York City show that in this setting spiritualism as a form of folk psychiatry retains its vitality and functions (Wakefield, 1959; Garrison, 1977; Harwood, 1977), and that it converges with the eclectic Christian, African, and West Indian religious practice of *santería*.

Assertions have been made that folk healers may be more in harmony with Hispanic views of mental illness than traditional therapists (Arenas et al., 1980) and that therapists and folk healers should work together (Abad et al., 1974) under some circumstances or whenever feasible (Bluestone and Purdy, 1977). Such proposals assume that folk healing practices are deeply and pervasively rooted in the culture, so that their incorporation into the clinical setting represents nothing more than the extension of indigenous culture into the official mental health system. But the question of how often and how pervasively folk healers are used and the attitudes of Hispanics toward folk healers has not been clearly answered, in particular with respect to Mexican Americans. Thus, where one study finds that most people would not use folk healers (Herrera and Sanchez, 1976; Keefe, 1978), another finds Mexican Americans willing to accept both drugs from a psychiatrist and herbal medicine from a healer (Castro, 1977). Or, folk healing may be a resource that is used when professional help is not available (Padilla et al., 1975); a treatment that may be used in conjunction with traditional therapy (Keefe and Casas, 1978); or a relatively unimportant factor (Karno and Edgerton, 1969). One reason offered for this mixed picture is that Mexican Americans may be ashamed of folk healing in the American context and will not admit that they have recourse to it (Vega, 1980). A second suggestion is that folk healing is primarily a lower class phenomenon in rural areas, and may be used less or discarded in urban and economically advantaged communities (Keefe and Casas, 1978). On the other hand, the literature on Puerto Ricans, as mentioned before, seems to indicate a widespread use of folk healing, although a more recent study of inner-city Puerto Ricans (Rodriguez, 1987) found that less than 5 percent of respondents reported consulting spiritualists. It should be noted that the use of both spiritualists and mental health professionals is not necessarily incompatible. Rogler and Hollingshead (1985) have noted that Puerto Ricans often intertwine their use of spiritualists with therapists.

In sum, the social organizations enmeshing Hispanics—the family, neighbors, and friends, the fictive coparent system, and indigenous folk healers—represent alternative resources for coping with emotional problems. To some researchers (Padilla et al., 1976), these resources represent the most potent explanation for the underutilization of mental health facilities. Our examination of underutilization as a research problem focusing on alternative resource theory has several implications. First, if we take the broader meaning of the concept of underutilization—high mental health need conjoined with low utilization—to be factually correct, then a crucial question is whether Hispanic informal social organizations have the strength necessary for coping with the psychological problems of its members. Is this strength being utilized to resolve or contain many of the Hispanics' psychological problems after they arise without resorting to professional mental health practitioners? However, it may be that despite such strength, the primary group structures are not capable of mitigating the impact of stresses arising from the Hispanics' disadvantaged and marginated status; thus, their high mental health needs. In examining the influence of alternative resources, therefore, three possible functions should be kept separate. The first function is the indigenous structure's capacity to keep psychological problems from arising. The second and third functions come into play once problems have arisen: the indigenous structure's capacity to treat or contain such problems and its capacity to refer afflicted individuals to professional mental health services. Finally, if the Hispanic family and other indigenous social groups contain, within their boundaries, emotional problems and provide emotional support once problems arise, such functions have important implications for the organization of mental health services in Hispanic communities. It would imply, as Valle (1980) suggests, that mental health facilities should actively promote the use of Hispanic community members as collaborating care providers.

The second explanation for the underutilization of mental health facilities is couched in terms of barriers which keep Hispanics away from such facilities. Two types of barriers, markedly distinct, have been posited to keep Hispanics away from mental health services: cultural and institutional barriers. We shall discuss cultural barriers first.

Cultural barriers may be found in subcultural values and beliefs which dispose those who identify with them to perceive emotional problems in such a way as not to seek professional services. One would expect that such perceptions, as well as the interpretations which inevitably are made of them, are subject to cultural variability. The findings on this issue, however, are mixed. Some studies find little difference between the ways Anglos and Mexican Americans perceive mental illness (Karno and Edgerton, 1969; Edgerton and Karno, 1971), whereas other studies indicate such differences (Newton, 1978; Padilla et al., 1975).

Some studies have identified specific folk beliefs about the nature of mental illness which may be linked to shunning professional help. In a study referred to previously, Rogler and Hollingshead (1985) examined Puerto Rican cultural conceptions of the *loco* or crazy person. To be crazy is a sharply defined stigma and means losing all socially valued attributes. Crazy persons are seen to behave in ways that are antithetical to the society's value system. The deviant behavior of the crazy person, therefore, is viewed in a moral context, thus causing the person to attempt to suppress or avoid divulging his or her symptoms. Unable to do so, the schizophrenic person is classified as crazy and, when punished for being a norm-breaker, he or she withdraws from customary social contacts. The study's data demonstrate that culturally defined labels of deviance associated with mental illness have a pronounced impact upon the afflicted person's help-seeking efforts, the treatment he or she receives in customary relations, and the deeply rooted reluctance to go to a psychiatric hospital which evokes the stigma of being crazy.

The influence of folk beliefs on the use of services has been of interest also to students of Mexican American behavior who have observed that Mexican Americans tend to delay mental health treatment because they do not classify symptoms as those of mental illness until they become severe (Fabrega et al., 1968) and that they view illness as a manifestation of weakness of character, and the need for treatment, as a disgraceful loss of pride (Newton, 1978). However, most research on folk beliefs among Mexican Americans has focused upon beliefs about physical illness rather than mental illness. Most of the studies find that acculturated Mexican Americans in urban settings do not subscribe to traditional views of physical illness and are more likely to consult physicians than folk healers (Castro et al., 1984; Farge, 1977; Keefe, 1981). One study (Karno and Edgerton, 1974) found no differences between Mexican Americans and Anglo Americans in their views about the causation of mental illness. In turn, a study of U.S. Puerto Ricans (Rodriguez, 1987) found no relationship between the extent of traditional folk beliefs and utilization.

Going beyond specific folk beliefs about mental illness, some studies have linked adherence to Hispanic values with the underutilization of mental health facilities. The cultural values mentioned in the literature are: *confianza* or the value of trust (Keefe, 1978); *personalismo* or trust in the immediate person, not the secondary institution (Keefe, 1978); *respeto* or the value of respect intrinsically owed to older persons (Abad et al., 1974; Bluestone and Purdy, 1977); *verguenza* and *orgullo* or the sense of shame and the value of pride (Romero, 1980); and *machismo* or the pride in manliness and its associated attributes (Abad et al., 1974). Other values are a part of this configuration, such as familism, fatalism, and orientation toward the present. The literature on utilization treats such values largely as descriptive, ethnographic categories to explain Hispanic underutilization. The underlying argument, however, is seldom made explicit: such values arise from and reinforce the interpersonal matrix of a primary group society based upon face-to-face intimate relationships. Hispanics adhering to such values, therefore, avoid or experience discomfort in their contacts with impersonal, second-ary, bureaucratic organizations such as mental health service agencies. Hence, they underutilize the service of these agencies. Presented in its sim-plest terms, this argument predicts underutilization or diminished contact with all bureaucratic services, not just mental health agencies. Plausible as the argument is because of its commendable use of elements in the ethnic culture, to our knowledge no single piece of research has sought to test di-rectly, and with appropriate controls, the relationship between varying de-grees of adherence to Hispanic beliefs and values, on one hand, and rates of utilization, on the other hand.

Several utilization studies subsume beliefs and values under the concept of acculturation—the process whereby the behaviors and attitudes of an immigrant group change towards the host society as a result of exposure to a different cultural system. In some studies, language use and preference are taken as the main indicator of acculturation. In others, generational sta-tus in relation to the original migration, number of years in the United States, ethnic self-identification, association with other ethnic groups, or a combination of these, are used as indicators. These studies generally have found that highly acculturated Hispanics are more likely to utilize services than their unacculturated counterparts (Chesney et al., 1982; Griffith and Villavicencio, 1985; Rodriguez, 1987). However, the studies raise questions about the extent to which education and income confound the effects of acculturation.

The literature also raises the possibility that acculturation influences uti-lization indirectly, through its effects on other factors believed to influence the use of mental health services. For example, Edgerton and Karno (1971) found that Mexican Americans who preferred to be interviewed in Span-ish—an indicator of lack of acculturation—were the most likely to adhere to traditional beliefs and perceptions regarding mental illness. The less ac-culturated were more likely than the acculturated to consider depression a more serious problem; they more often considered that mental illness is inherited and more often viewed prayer as an effective mode of treatment. It is not clear from this or other studies whether acculturation-influenced mental health beliefs in turn influence Hispanics' disposition to use mental health professionals.

Now that we have examined the influences of Hispanic culture and indig-enous social organizations on utilization, the links between these factors should become more explicit. For example, members of an extended family are more likely to provide emotional support to a troubled person when all share cultural beliefs distinctly separate from the beliefs of the professional mental health system. Nevertheless, subcultural beliefs and indigenous social organization are conceptually distinct, and each could act independently to influence help-seeking. Friedson's typology (1961, 1970) of lay referral systems makes this clear. The lay referral system should be understood as an interpersonal system that diagnoses and provides treatment. Friedson's typology is based upon the combination of two elements: (1) the congruence or incongruence between the lay and the professional culture according to elements we have described earlier, such as language, values, and the perceptions of illness and appropriate treatments; and (2) the structure of the lay referral system which may be loose and truncated or cohesive and extended. If the structure is loose and truncated, the persons are left on their own or they consult only with members of their immediate families. If it is cohesive and extended, the persons have available to them a large number of people—inside and outside the family—with whom to consult. The combination of the elements yields four types of lay referral systems. For our purposes, the most important type is the one which combines an incongruity between lay referral culture and professional medical culture, on the one hand, and a lay referral structure which is extended and cohesive, on the other hand. In this type, the help-seeking effort occurs as a sequence of steps through the extended and cohesive lay referral system (the indigenous social organization), before contact is made with the professional system. Delays in contacting the professional system or the avoidance of the system are due to the availability of an extended and cohesive group of help-givers, and to the fact that membership in such a group reinforces the cultural incompatibility between the lay and professional system.

Hispanics' efforts to cope with psychological problems appear to fit this type of lay referral system, as is evident in the literature we have reviewed, and in other literature as well (Suchman, 1964). Not only do they fit in a descriptive sense, but the predictions which derive from being so classified conform to the Hispanics' low utilization rates of mental health services. The expectation is that when the lay referral systems (or the indigenous social structures) are socially or structurally intertwined with the mental health system and the cultural differences between the two are thus reduced, utilization rates among Hispanics will increase. In this situation, the professional system reaches out to the cohesive and extended lay referral system to increase its accessibility and to assimilate elements of indigenous or lay culture in the interest of attracting persons to use its services.

Acculturation has also been linked to the extent of social support offered by family and friends, the major link with underutilization posited by alternative resource theory. Griffith and Villavicencio (1985) found that acculturated Mexican Americans had larger networks of family and friends, more contacts with network members, and relied more on them than the unacculturated. Although they do not report whether this relationship influenced psychological distress or utilization, in another article based on the same data, Griffith (1984) reported that the acculturated had fewer anxiety symptoms but more symptoms of psychosocial dysfunction. Since their work did not examine the interrelationship between acculturation, social supports, and utilization, their findings bear only tangentially upon the assumptions of alternative resource and cultural barrier theories. However, Rodriguez's (1987) findings are pertinent here, since his study found that, among psychologically distressed Puerto Ricans, having an extensive and active network of family and friends was associated with increased use of mental health services, regardless of acculturation. In sum, the studies which have examined the influences on utilization of Hispanic indigenous social organization and Hispanic culture are too few to provide a pattern of conclusions about the interrelationship among these factors. However, they have brought forth interesting hypotheses about the complex ways in which social networks and acculturation may influence mental health and the utilization of mental health services.

We have distinguished between alternative resource theory, which points to the existence of alternative sources of mental health care, and cultural barrier theory, which points to the existence of Hispanic cultural values and beliefs which act as impediments to the use of mental health facilities. We now turn to a different aspect of barrier theory—institutional barriers— which posits that characteristics of the mental health system keep Hispanics from using mental health services. Institutional barrier theory states that there are structural incongruities between the characteristics of Hispanic culture and those of the mental health system, not the least problem being the prejudice and discrimination leveled at Hispanics. The theory does not see Hispanic culture or indigenous social organizations as an obstacle to use of professional care. On the contrary, it assumes that Hispanics want to seek professional help, but are rebuffed by the way in which mental health care is organized. What are the structural incongruities in the organization of professional mental health care, and how do they keep Hispanics from using facilities? As with other aspects of utilization theory, the literature contains many hypothetical assertions, but little confirmatory research. We begin by enumerating the types of institutional barriers which have been hypothesized and then assess the research addressing the theory.

The most commonly cited institutional obstacle to utilization is the lack of Spanish-speaking, bicultural professionals in mental health facilities

(Abad et al., 1975; Keefe and Casas, 1980; Levine and Padilla, 1980). The argument is simple: one can hardly expect Hispanics to seek help in facilities where help-providers cannot communicate effectively with them and have little or no understanding of Hispanic folk beliefs and the primary group norms of interaction cited above in our discussion of cultural barriers.

In addition to cultural and perceptual differences, socioeconomic differences between the Hispanic patient and therapist may result in underutilization. The difficulty of middle-class therapists in working with lower-class patients and with patients who are not youthful, attractive, verbal, intelligent, and successful is mentioned frequently (Hollingshead and Redlich, 1958; Lorion, 1973, 1974). Since the values of patients can affect utilization of services, so the values of therapists can affect accessibility to those services (Padilla et al., 1975). It is the middle-class character and values of the entire mental health movement that Reissman and Scribner (1965) see as one of three major barriers to proper mental health utilization by the poor (the others being fear of institutionalization and stigmatic attitudes toward mental illness). When we consider that blacks have higher rates of utilization than Hispanics, the caution that culture, class, and language interact to cause low Hispanic utilization appears to be well taken (Padilla et al., 1975).

The search for explanations for such complicated interactions should not lead to the neglect of more simple explanations, such as geographic inaccessibility or lack of income. Mental health clinics are often located in schools of medicine or universities outside the Hispanic community (Karno and Edgerton, 1969; Padilla et al., 1975; Keefe, 1978). However, even this explanation becomes complicated in the light of survey reports which show that Mexican Americans aware of nearby clinic locations still have low rates of utilization (Padilla et al., 1976). Perhaps this is linked to the alleged lack of attention personnel in mental health facilities give to the characteristics of their patients (Karno, 1966), or to blatant racism in patient selection and treatment (Vega, 1980). With respect to income as a barrier, some observers note that the advent of Medicaid and Medicare has made health services more accessible to the poor (Veroff et al., 1981), but it has also been observed that these services are available only to the lowest income strata, and not to those making low-to-modest incomes (Davis and Schoen, 1978).

In sum, institutional barrier theory focuses upon the incongruities and tensions between the collective attributes of Hispanics as actual or potential mental health clients and the procedures and characteristics of the mental health agency system. Accordingly, explanations for underutilization have been sought in the failures of mental health organizations to adjust their services to Hispanic language, values, folk beliefs, and characteristics. Barrier theory predicts that when such incongruities diminish over time, utilization rates increase; or that in those areas where such incongruities are weak or nonexistent, utilization rates are comparatively higher. Does research verify these predictions? Case studies of individual facilities that modified the structure of their services to make them more attractive to Hispanics suggest that the predictions of institutional barrier theory are correct. Let us examine the evidence from such studies.

The work of Bloom (1975) is relevant to the first prediction that utilization rates increase over time when mental health facilities address structural incongruities. Bloom found that Hispanics in Pueblo, Colorado, went from being underrepresented in regard to inpatient admissions in 1960 to being overrepresented in such admissions in 1970, a finding which also may reflect higher mental health needs among Mexican Americans. The increase was attributed to an improved image of the mental health system, an increase in Chicano staff, and the increased availability of financial aid programs. Flores (1978) reported increases in utilization rates as a result of similar interventions in the East Los Angeles Mental Health Service, and Fischman et al. (1983) described similar results in California's San Mateo County.

Rodriguez (1986) demonstrated a link between the creation of a bilingual/bicultural professional staff and the increase in Hispanic clients in a study of a community mental health center located in a predominantly Puerto Rican area of the South Bronx. In order to increase the utilization of aftercare services by chronically mentally ill Hispanics, the center hired a bilingual staff to conduct outreach among Bronx psychiatric facility patients and their relatives and provided services in Spanish. The aftercare service was thus able to increase Hispanic representation among its clients from 40 to 49 percent over a six-month period.

Research by Treviño et al. (1979) is relevant to the second prediction deriving from barrier theory, namely, that Hispanic utilization rates are high in areas where structural incongruities do not exist. Treviño's research took place in Laredo, Texas, an area predominantly inhabited by Mexican Americans and with a mental health center in which structural barriers had been minimized. The mental health center had a bilingual Mexican American staff indigenous to the area and utilized a sliding-fee scale in charging for services, but never refused service because of inability to pay. These features of the community mental health center reduced language, cultural, social class, and economic barriers. Because the city of Laredo is predominantly Mexican American, the effect of being a member of a minority group was also reduced. The researchers found that for the majority of census tracts, Mexican Americans met or exceeded their expected utilization of mental health services as determined by the ethnic composition of each tract. The study's conclusions are instructive: ". . . underrepresentation of Mexican American clients in community mental health centers reflects barriers to utilization rather than a lower need for service . . ." (p.334).

Although these case studies support institutional barrier theory, to date no research based upon large samples has tested the hypothesized relationship between organizational characteristics and underutilization of mental health services. When it is conducted, the research could well demonstrate such a relationship, as is suggested by aggregate data studies of services for the elderly. Holmes et al. (1979) and Snyder (1981), in studies using counties as units of observation, found that characteristics such as the percentage of minorities on staff and the extent of agency location in minority neighborhoods predicted the proportions of minority elderly receiving services. Some studies have addressed the issue of institutional barriers by observing the behavior and attitudes of help-seekers. Because institutional barriers are attributes of organizations, research based on observations of individuals can infer the existence of institutional barriers only indirectly. The assumption is that if certain organizational characteristics present obstacles to utilization, individuals holding negative perceptions of the organizations' services should be expected not to make use of these services. Rodriguez (1987) found that persons with the most negative views of services in the catchment area were the ones using mental health services, but this suggests that use shapes attitudes. Keefe and Casas (1980) note the lack of a relationship between utilization and perceptions of agencies in their study of Mexican Americans, and Stefl and Prosperi (1985) note the same in a study of utilization among a rural non-minority sample.

The studies cited above cannot be considered to disconfirm barrier theory. However, their findings bring up critical questions about perceptions of institutional characteristics by Hispanics and other minorities. Are attributes of mental health facilities most evident to the help-seeker after he or she comes into contact with the facility, i.e., after the successful completion of a help-seeking sequence? Making note of the lack of a relationship between perceptions of services and underutilization, Barrera (1978) has suggested that such perceptions may be the result of receiving inadequate services rather than a cause of underutilization. If this view is correct, negative perceptions of facilities may discourage help-seeking only after repeated unsuccessful attempts to obtain adequate services. On the other hand, since these studies measure perceptions of services *post hoc,* it may be that utilizers originally had more positive perceptions of the services they sought. The mechanisms by which institutional barriers are perceived may be more complex than what is implied by existing studies based on cross-sectional surveys.

Now that we have examined research findings bearing upon the major explanations of Hispanic underutilization, the need for research examining the interrelationships among factors relevant to these explanations should be apparent. Is the organizational character of the mental health services system an obstacle to utilization which is superimposed on other obstacles imbedded in Hispanic culture? Do institutional barriers dovetail with the tendencies of Hispanic social networks to provide alternatives to professional care, as posited by alternative resource theory? The studies reviewed suggest these questions, but they cannot answer them. We turn now to considerations of how future research should address these questions.

To address the issues we have discussed, research relevant to the second phase must include five components: (1) epidemiological data on the true prevalence of psychological distress in the Hispanic population designated for research; (2) measures of the degree to which Hispanic respondents are integrated into the indigenous social organizations serving as alternative mental health resources; (3) measures of the Hispanic respondents' degree of acculturation; (4) direct measures of the organizational features of the available mental health service facilities; and (5) Hispanic utilization rates in the available mental health facilities. If research does not examine the first four components in order to understand the fifth—utilization, the results will inevitably be ambiguous. For example, underutilization in a logical sense could be characterized by low need, the existence of strong alternative resources, and the absence of barriers. Or, underutilization could be characterized by a high need, weak alternative resources, and formidable barriers. It is only by viewing the interrelationships among the first four factors through comprehensively organized research that we can begin to narrow the margin of ambiguity.

These are the main features of the two research problems relevant to the second phase of the framework: the extent to which Hispanics, in relation to their needs, underutilize mental health facilities and the interrelationships among the factors which explain such underutilization. Now that we have outlined the major hypothesized factors and their interrelationship it is appropriate to introduce time as an additional factor, thus conceiving a help-seeking behavior as an attempt over time to cope with psychological distress. Practically all of the cross-sectional studies discussed here reveal a surprisingly consistent neglect of the time dimension in the human effort to cope with a mental health problem. It is surprising because the effort to cope, the indicated target of research, is clearly and unmistakeably a social process bound by time; yet time plays virtually no role in the research. Thus, we do not believe there is any possibility of reconciling differences in the findings of the literature reported here or of attaining consistency in the findings of future research unless the research topic is framed as a temporal process in which mental health problems, alternative resources, and barriers influence each other as they influence contacts with the professional mental health system. Only through the introduction of time as a variable is it possible to determine, for example, whether the indigenous social organizations contain emotional problems or whether the help-seeker's relation to the organizations changes once emotional problems emerge; whether acculturation influences the emergence of emotional problems, or Hispanics' disposition to contact mental health professionals, or both. To adequately capture the process requires a research program involving repeated measures over time of the five components outlined above.

The need for epidemiologically-based panel studies, however, should not obscure the need for qualitative research to develop hypotheses about the most likely interrelationships among these factors. This research would seek to identify the tangible efforts Hispanics make over time to cope with mental distress. The research would delineate successive contacts with indigenous social organizations and professionals as they attempt to cope with mental distress. The research could be oriented retrospectively by focusing upon clients who have already made their first contact with mental health agencies, or preferably, prospectively, by identifying the first experience of mental distress and then tracking the coping effort. The concept of pathways to the mental health system (Hollingshead and Redlich, 1958) provides a useful orientation to the research because it calls attention to successive contacts from one indigenous social organization to the next or to several at the same time before or while the agency system is contacted. The properties of the pathway are likely to vary in number, order, and variety of organizations contacted, and in the duration of the contacts. Barrier theory fits the approach being proposed by providing hypotheses to explain how the help-seeking effort described by the pathway is either suppressed or expedited in moving toward contact with the mental health agency system.

Summary

We have identified two research problems relevant to Phase Two of our conceptual framework which concerns help-seeking efforts by Hispanics to alleviate psychological distress. The first research problem is the extent to which Hispanics underutilize mental health facilities when their admission rates are weighed against their mental illness prevalence rates. The second research problem concerns the need to examine the interrelationships among factors relevant to the major theories of Hispanic underutilization. In examining findings from studies addressing these theories, we have shown that alternative resource theory and cultural and institutional barriers theory can be integrated to provide a more dynamic and comprehensive framework for research focusing upon the clinical services framework's second phase. The use of such a framework should capture more accurately and extensively the Hispanic experience of mental health service utilization, and thus improve mental health policy and practice affecting the Hispanic community.

References

Abad, V., Ramos, J. and Boyce, E. (1974). A model for delivery of mental health services to Spanish-speaking minorities. *American Journal of Orthopsychiatry* 44(4): 584-595.

Alers, J.O. (1978). *Puerto Ricans and Health: Findings from New York City.* New York: Hispanic Research Center, Fordham University (Monograph No. 1).

Arenas, S., Cross, H. and Willard, W. (1980). Curanderos and mental health professionals: A comparative study on perceptions of psychopathology. *Hispanic Journal of Behavioral Sciences* 2(4): 407-421.

Bachrach, L. (1975). *Utilization of State and County Mental Hospitals by Spanish Americans in 1972.* NIMH Division of Biometry, Statistical Note 116, DHEW Publication No. (ADM) 75-158. Washington, D.C.: U.S. Government Printing Office.

Barrera, M. (1978). Mexican American mental health service utilization: A critical examination of some proposed variables. *Community Mental Health Journal* 14(1): 35-45.

Bloom, B. (1975). *Changing Patterns of Psychiatric Care.* New York: Human Sciences Press.

Bluestone, H. and Purdy, B. (1977). Psychiatric services to Puerto Rican patients in the Bronx. In E.R. Padilla and A.M. Padilla (Eds.), *Transcultural Psychiatry: An Hispanic Perspective.* Los Angeles: Spanish-Speaking Mental Health Center, University of California (Monograph No. 4).

Brameld, T. (1959). *The Remaking of a Culture: Life and Education in Puerto Rico.* New York: Harper.

Castro, F.G. (1977). Level of acculturation and related considerations in psychotherapy with Spanish-speaking/surnamed clients. Los Angeles: Spanish-Speaking Mental Health Research Center, University of California (Occasional Paper No. 3).

Castro, F.G., Furth, P. and Karlow, H. (1984). The health beliefs of Mexican, Mexican-American, and Anglo-American women. *Hispanic Journal of Behavioral Sciences* 6(4): 365-383.

Chesney, A.P., Chavira, J.A., Hall, R.P. and Giary, H.E. (1982). Barriers to medical care of Mexican Americans: The role of social class, acculturation, and social isolation. *Medical Care* 20(9): 883-892.

Cochran, T.C. (1959). *The Puerto Rican Businessman: A Study in Cultural Change.* Philadelphia: University of Pennsylvania Press.

Davis, K. and Schoen, C. (1978). *Health and the War on Poverty.* Washington, D.C.: Brookings Institution.

Edgerton, R.B. and Karno, M. (1971). Mexican-American bilingualism and the perception of mental illness. *Archives of General Psychiatry* 24: 286-290.

Fabrega, H., Jr., Swartz, J.D. and Wallace, C.A. (1968). Ethnic differences in psychopathology II—Specific differences with emphasis on a Mexican American group. *Psychiatric Research* 6(3): 221-235.

Farge, E.J. (1977). A review of findings from "three generations" of Chicano health care behavior. *Social Sciences Quarterly* 58: 407-411.

Fischman, G., Fraticelli B., Newman, D.E. and Sampson, L.M. (1983). Day-treatment programs for the Spanish-speaking: A response to underutilization. *International Journal of Social Psychiatry* 29(3): 215-219.

Fitzpatrick, J.P. (1971). *Puerto Rican Americans: The Meaning of Migration to the Mainland.* Englewood Cliffs, N.J.: Prentice Hall.

Fitzpatrick, J.P. and Gould, R. (1968). *Mental Health Needs of Spanish-Speaking Children in the New York Area.* New York: Institute for Social Research, Fordham University.

Flores, J.L. (1978). The utilization of a community mental health service by Mexican Americans. *International Journal of Social Psychiatry* 24: 271-275.

Friedson, E. (1961). *Patients' Views of Medical Practice. A Study of Subscribers to a Prepaid Medical Plan in the Bronx.* New York: Russell Sage Foundation.

Friedson, E. (1970). *Profession of Medicine. A Study of the Sociology of Applied Knowledge.* New York: Dodd, Mead and Co.

Garrison, V. (1977). Doctor, espiritista or psychiatrist? Health seeking behavior in a Puerto Rican neighborhood of New York City. *Medical Anthropology* 1(2): 165-180.

Griffith, J. (1984). Relationship between acculturation and psychological impairment in adult Mexican Americans. *Hispanic Journal of Behavioral Sciences* 5(4): 431-459.

Griffith, J. and Villavicencio, S. (1985). Relationship among acculturation, sociodemographic characteristics and social support in Mexican American adults. *Hispanic Journal of Behavioral Sciences* 7(1): 75-92.

Harwood, A. (1977). *Rx: Spiritist as Needed: A Study of a Puerto Rican Community Mental Health Resource.* New York: Wiley and Sons.

Herrera, A.E. and Sanchez, V.C. (1976). Behaviorally oriented group therapy: A successful application in the treatment of low-income Spanish-speaking clients (pp. 73-84). In M.R. Miranda (Ed.), *Psychotherapy with the Spanish Speaking: Issues in Research and Service Delivery.* Los Angeles: Spanish-Speaking Mental Health Research Center, University of California (Monograph No. 3).

Hollingshead, A.B. and Redlich, F.C. (1958). *Social Class and Mental Illness.* New York: Wiley and Sons.

Holmes, D., Holmes, M., Steinbach, L. and Hausner, T. (1979). The use of community based services in long-term care by older minority persons. *Gerontologist* 19(4).

Hoppe, S. and Heller, P. (1975). Alienation, familism and the utilization of health services by Mexican Americans. *Journal of Health and Social Behavior* 16: 304-314.

Karno, M. (1966). The enigma of ethnicity in a psychiatric clinic. *Archives of General Psychiatry* 14: 516-520.

Karno, M. and Edgerton, R.B. (1969). Perception of mental illness in a Mexican American community. *Archives of General Psychiatry* 20: 233-238.

Karno, M. and Edgerton, R.B. (1974). Some folk beliefs about mental illness: A reconsideration. *International Journal of Social Psychiatry* 20: 292-296.

Keefe, S.E. (1978). Why Mexican Americans underutilize mental health clinics: Facts and fallacy (pp. 91-108). In J.M. Casas and S.E. Keefe (Eds.), *Family and Mental Health in the Mexican American Community.* Los Angeles: Spanish-Speaking Mental Health Research Center, University of California (Monograph No. 7).

Keefe, S.E. (1979). Mexican Americans' underutilization of mental health clinics: An evaluation of suggested explanations. *Hispanic Journal of Behavioral Sciences* 1(2): 93-115.

Keefe, S.E. (1981). Folk medicine among urban Mexican Americans: Cultural persistence, change, and displacement. *Hispanic Journal of Behavioral Sciences* 3(1): 41-58.

Keefe, S.E., Padilla, A. and Carlos, M. (1978). The Mexican American extended family as an emotional support system (pp.49-68). In J.M. Casas and S.E. Keefe (Eds.), *Family and Mental Health in the Mexican American Community.* Los Angeles: Spanish-Speaking Mental Health Research Center, University of California (Monograph No. 7).

Keefe, S.E. and Casas, J.M. (1978). Family and mental health among Mexican Americans: Some considerations for mental health services (pp.1-24). In J.M. Casas and S.E. Keefe (Eds.), *Family and Mental Health in the Mexican American Community.* Los Angeles: Spanish-Speaking Mental Health Research Center, University of California (Monograph No. 7).

Keefe, S.E. and Casas, J.M. (1980). Mexican Americans and mental health: A selected review and recommendations for mental health service delivery. *American Journal of Community Psychology* 8(3).

Levine, E.S. and Padilla, A.M. (1980). *Crossing Cultures in Therapy: Pluralistic Counseling for the Hispanic.* Monterrey, California: Brooks/Cole Publishing Co.

Lopez, S. (1981). Mexican American usage of mental health facilities: Underutilization reconsidered (pp.139-164). In A. Baron, Jr. (Ed.), *Explorations in Chicano Psychology.* New York: Praeger.

Lorion, R.P. (1973). Socioeconomic status and traditional treatment approaches reconsidered. *Psychological Bulletin* 79(4): 263-270.

Lorion, R.P. (1974). Patient and therapist variables in the treatment of low-income patients. *Psychological Bulletin* 81(6): 344-354.

Mann, E. and Salvo, J. (1985). Characteristics of new Hispanic immigrants to New York City: A comparison of Puerto Rican and non-Puerto Rican Hispanics. Hispanic Research Center, Fordham University, *Research Bulletin* 8(1-2) January-April.

Mintz, S.W. (1956). Cañamelar: The subculture of a rural sugar plantation proletariat. In J.H. Steward et al. (Eds.). *The People of Puerto Rico: A Study in Social Anthropology.* Urbana: University of Illinois Press.

National Institute of Mental Health (1976a). *Services to the Mentally Disabled of Metropolitan Community Mental Health Catchment Areas.* Series B, No. 10, DHEW Publication No. (ADM) 76-373. Washington, D.C.: U.S. Government Printing Office.

National Institute of Mental Health (1976b). *Services to the Mentally Disabled of Selected Catchment Areas in Eastern New York State and New York City.* DHEW Publication No. (ADM) 76-372. Washington, D.C.: U.S. Government Printing Office.

National Institute of Mental Health (1980). *Hispanic Americans and Mental Health Facilities: A Comparison of Hispanic, Black and White Admissions to Selected Mental Health Facilities, 1975.* Series CN, No. 3, DHHS Publication No. (ADM) 80-1006. Washington, D.C.: U.S. Government Printing Office.

Newton, F. (1978). The Mexican American emic system of mental illness: An exploratory study (pp.69-90). In J.M. Casas and S.E. Keefe (Eds.), *Family and Mental Health in the Mexican American Community.* Los Angeles: Spanish-Speaking Mental Health Research Center, University of California (Monograph No. 7).

New York State Office of Mental Health (1982). *Survey of Patient Characteristics, 1981.* Albany, N.Y.: NYSOMH.

Padilla, A.M., Ruiz, R.A. and Alvarez, R. (1975). Community mental health services for the Spanish-speaking/surnamed population. *American Psychologist* 30 (September): 892-905.

Padilla, A.M., Carlos, M. and Keefe, S.E. (1976). Mental health utilization by Mexican Americans (pp.9-20). In M. Miranda (Ed.), *Psychotherapy with the Spanish-Speaking: Issues in Research and Service Delivery.* Los Angeles: Spanish-Speaking Mental Health Research Center, University of California (Monograph No. 3).

Reissman, F. and Scribner, S. (1965). The underutilization of mental health services by workers and low-income groups: Causes and cures. *American Journal of Psychiatry* 121 (February): 798-801.

Roberts, L. and Stefani, R.L. (1949). *Patterns of Living in Puerto Rican Families.* Rio Piedras: Editorial Universitaria.

Rodriguez, O. (1986). Overcoming barriers to services among chronically mentally ill Hispanics: Lessons from the Project COPA evaluation. *Research Bulletin* 9(1), Hispanic Research Center, Fordham University, Bronx, New York.

Rodriguez, O. (1987). *Hispanics and Human Services: Help-Seeking in the Inner City.* Bronx, N.Y.: Hispanic Research Center, Fordham University (Monograph No. 14).

Rogler, L.H. (1978). Help patterns, the family, and mental health: Puerto Ricans in the United States. *International Migration Review* 12(2): 248-259.

Rogler, L.H. and Hollingshead, A.B. (1960). Algunas observaciones sobre el espiritismo y las enfermedades mentales entre puertorriqueños de clase baja. *Revista de Ciencias Sociales* 4(1): 141-150.

Rogler, L.H. and Hollingshead, A.B. (1961). The Puerto Rican spiritist as psychiatrist. *American Journal of Sociology* 87(1): 17-21.

Rogler, L.H. and Hollingshead, A.B. (1985). *Trapped: Puerto Rican Families and Schizophrenia,* 3rd ed. Maplewood, N.J.: Waterfront Press.

Rogler, L.H. and Cooney, R.S. (1984). *Puerto Rican Families in New York City: Intergenerational Processes.* Maplewood, N.J.: Waterfront Press (Hispanic Research Center Monograph No. 11).

Romero, J.T. (1980). Hispanic support systems: Health-mental health promotion strategies. In R. Valle and W. Vega (Eds.), *Hispanic Natural Support Systems: Mental Health Promotion Perspectives.* State of California: Department of Mental Health.

Snyder, C. (Ed.) (1981). *Maximizing Utilization of Community-Based Services by the Minority Elderly.* New York: Community Council of Greater New York.

Stefl, M.E. and Prosperi, D.G. (1985). Barriers to mental health service utilization. *Community Mental Health Journal* 21(3): 167-178.

Suchman, E.A. (1964). Sociomedical variations among ethnic groups. *American Journal of Sociology* 70: 319-331.

Treviño, F.M., Bruhn, J.G. and Bunce, H. III (1979). Utilization of community mental health services in a Texas-Mexico border city. *Social Science and Medicine* 13(3A): 331-334.

Tumin, M.M. and Feldman, A.S. (1961). *Social Class and Social Change in Puerto Rico.* New Jersey: Princeton University Press.

U.S. Bureau of the Census (1963). *Census of Population: 1960. Subject Reports. Final Report PC(2)-ID, Puerto Ricans in the United States.* Washington, D.C.: U.S. Government Printing Office.

U.S. Bureau of the Census (1973). *Census of Population: 1970. Subject Reports. Final Report PC(2)-IE, Puerto Ricans in the United States.* Washington, D.C.: U.S. Government Printing Office.

U.S. Bureau of the Census (1980). *Census of Population: 1980. Subject Reports. Final Report PC (2) 1F, Puerto Ricans in the United States.* Washington, D.C.: U.S. Government Printing Office.

Valle, R. (1980). A natural resource system for health-mental health promotion to Latino/Hispano populations (pp.35-44). In R. Valle and W. Vega (Eds.) *Hispanic Natural Support Systems: Mental Health Promotion Perspectives.* California: State Department of Mental Health.

Vega, W. (1980). Mental health research and North American Hispanic populations: A review and a proposed research strategy (pp. 3-14). In R. Valle and W. Vega (Eds.), *Hispanic Natural Support Systems: Mental Health Promotion Perspectives.* California: State Department of Mental Health.

Veroff, J., Kulka, R.A. and Donovan, E. (1981). *Mental Health in America. Patterns of Help-Seeking from 1957 to 1976.* New York: Basic Books.

Wakefield, D. (1959). *Island in the City: The World of Spanish Harlem.* Boston: Houghton Mifflin.

Wolf, K.L. (1952). Growing up and its price in three Puerto Rican subcultures. *Psychiatry* 15: 401-433.

Chapter 4

Phase Three: Evaluation of Mental Health

Ever since she was a child on a farm in Puerto Rico, Mrs. Maria Mercado has had frequent and vivid dreams. But it was not until she married her third husband that the dreams became nightmares. It began when her husband, a practicing spiritualist medium, brought three black men to their apartment to conduct a spiritualist session. The men announced that evil spirits had invaded her soul, an interpretation repeated in subsequent sessions. Her relatives fully agreed with the interpretations. One of the most revolting dreams to her was that of being sexually assaulted by black men. During childhood, her father told her that black men were evil and filthy, and she herself felt degraded at being identified by the family as the darkest of the thirteen children. To her, black men in her nightmares are evil spirits. Mrs. Mercado knows that dreams are dreams, but from spiritualism she knows that the dreams contain truth: "All dreams are revelations."

She has experienced and recognizes a repeated pattern in her life: whenever she separates from a loved person—in particular, her two sons and one grandchild—she immediately feels anxious and depressed, loses her appetite, and becomes nervous. Then is when the nightmares come to torment her sleep. Most of the time, however, Mrs. Mercado follows a daily round of intense social activities, giving advice to her relatives and friends, contacting and counseling her sons and grandchild, and sending money to relatives in Puerto Rico. She is very proud of the fact that on her own she raised her two sons and one grandson in Spanish Harlem and not one of them is addicted to drugs or has had criminal involvements. The three are employed and completely self-sufficient.

After one experience of separation from a loved one, feeling dejected, anxious, and crying, she was put in touch with a local community mental health center. The intake diagnostic impression by the non-Hispanic physician, referring to her "superstitious and spiritist cultural background," states that she suffers from schizophrenia. The diagnostic impression in her clinical records has not been superceded by a more definitive diagnosis. After three intensive interviews with Mrs. Mercado, a trained Hispanic interviewer observed: "There is a gentle manner about her. She was soft-spoken, in full command of the Spanish language, very articulate, calm, extremely pleasant and friendly. One would hardly suspect that Mrs. Mercado is mentally ill."

* * *

The third phase begins when the psychologically distressed person reaches a formal mental health setting and the process of mental health evaluation takes place. The psychologically distressed person's early contact with a mental health agency is likely to be diagnostic in nature, whether the assessment performed is formal or informal, brief or intensive. The procedure might include a mental status examination upon intake into the mental health facility; that is, an interview in which the client's presenting symptoms, contact with reality, and psychosocial history are disclosed. In addition, psychological tests might be administered, such as an intelligence test, a projective personality technique, or a paper-and-pencil personality inventory, along with a neurological screening device to probe for possible organic disorder. Results of the testing are evaluated in the context of the initial interview data and the client's psychosocial history, and at the end of this process a psychodiagnosis is formulated, a treatment plan is recommended, and a disposition of the case is rendered.

The question of whether the instruments used in psychological assessment, and even the interview process itself, are culturally biased has been hotly debated for many years. Such polemics acquired additional momentum in the early 1950's and 1960's with attention focusing upon the normative performance deficit of blacks on standardized intelligence tests and subsequent, largely unsuccessful attempts to develop so-called culture-free and culture-fair intelligence tests. The controversy reached its boiling point in the late 1960's when an emphasis was placed upon genetic explanations of normative differences. More recently, similar polemics have been rekindled by reports of higher prevalence rates of mental disorder and psychiatric symptomatology for Hispanics than for Anglo-Americans, as discussed in Chapter 2, and by the incisive scrutiny of cultural and language factors involved in personality test performance and behavior during a psychiatric interview.

This scenario of the assessment and diagnostic process and the attendant concerns in clinical practice with Hispanics pose two critical research problems in Phase Three of the framework. The first research problem concerns questions regarding cultural bias toward Hispanics in psychological tests which have been conceived, standardized, and validated in English with a non-minority, middle-class perspective. The second research problem concerns factors influencing the accuracy of clinical judgment of psychopathology and diagnosis in a psychiatric interview when the client is a bilingual Hispanic. In this chapter we shall consider the propriety of administering standardized psychological tests to Hispanics and the sociocultural dynamics of the psychiatric interview. We address the first research problem by commenting on the literature on test bias—limiting our discussion to the personality testing of Hispanics—and on efforts to develop and adapt personality tests for valid assessment of Hispanic clients. Then we turn to the second research problem on the influence of bilingualism and biculturalism on clinical judgment of psychopathology and diagnosis. Finally, the chapter concludes with some general observations about the current status of the two research problems, needs which should be addressed in future research, and the integration of the two problems in the context of the broader issue of how to achieve accurate mental health evaluations of Hispanic clients.

Personality Assessment of Hispanics

The application of psychological tests that have been standardized on non-minority, English-speaking populations to examinees who are non-native English speakers from different cultural backgrounds has been a controversy for over forty years (Olmedo, 1981). On one side of this controversy is the viewpoint that examinees' variations in English-language proficiency and cultural background are potential sources of distortion of observed test behavior, i.e., something other than the attributes that psychological assessment is intended to reveal is at issue (e.g., Malgady et al., 1987). The other side of the controversy argues that distorsion must first be empirically demonstrated, since it has not been unequivocally established in the domain of personality testing (e.g., Lopez, in press). Whether standardized tests should be considered innocent of bias until proven guilty will be discussed later in this chapter. Now we shall examine both sides of the controversy.

Psychological assessment typically involves a comparison of the behavior or performance of the examinee with that of others in a normative group. A Hispanic examinee may appear at the lower end of non-minority group norms, leading a clinician to infer the presence of pathology, yet be within or close to the average range for his or her own ethnic group. The impact of such misinterpretation of test performance on people's lives can be dramatic: as Reschly (1981), Garcia (1977), and McClelland (1973) show, a disproportionate number of ethnic minority children are classified as mentally retarded and emotionally disturbed. Similarly, Levine and Padilla (1980) list a number of personality tests on which Hispanics' profiles differ from the normative status of other ethnic groups. They conclude that cultural ideology and acculturation may influence responses on objective personality inventories and that open-ended projective tests tap personality traits as they vary with the cultural and social milieu. Even on open-ended tasks where a clinician does not make use of an explicit norm group, such as in an interview or informal projective assessment, an examinee is implicitly compared with a generalized view of a healthy person. The more the clinical impression of the examinee diverges from the clinician's own view of normal, the more pathological the examinee is judged. Hence the question of what frame of reference is being used, whether derived from standardized norms or from subtle clinical impressions, is of the utmost importance for the accurate assessment of Hispanics, since norms have meaning only if they are appropriate for the individual under consideration. It is not surprising, then, that the minority assessment literature gives a prominent place to differential normative performance as an issue of test bias and to the question of whether norms need to be developed separately for specific ethnic groups.

Perhaps the most comprehensive self-report personality inventory widely used for clinical assessment is the Minnesota Multiphasic Personality Inventory (MMPI), which has spawned multilingual translations. Prewitt-Diaz et al. (1984) provide a brief history of Spanish translations of the MMPI, beginning with early translations for Cubans (Paz, 1952) and Puerto Ricans (Bernal et al., 1959—cited in Prewitt-Diaz et al., 1984), a later adaptation of the Puerto Rican version to Mexican Americans (Nuñez, 1967, 1968), and other versions used in Spain (Echevarria et al., 1969) and in Chile (Risetti, 1981).

However, the MMPI does not emerge unscathed in the test bias literature, which focuses primarily on black-white comparisons. There is a rift of professional opinion on whether separate norms are required as a function of ethnicity (Gynther and Green, 1980; Pritchard and Rosenblatt, 1980). In a review we undertook of the MMPI literature on the theme of ethnicity over a ten-year period (1975-1985), we located 38 articles in psychology journals, only six of which discussed whether norms for Hispanics differed from those for whites or blacks. One study concluded that separate Hispanic MMPI norms are not necessary—on the basis of a sample of 11 Hispanics (Page and Bozlee, 1982). Four of the remaining studies reported significant differences between Hispanics and other ethnic groups and between English and Spanish test forms on selected MMPI scales (Fuller and Malony, 1984; Holland, 1979; McCreary and Padilla, 1977; McGill, 1980). The remaining study (Prewitt-Diaz et al., 1984) presented a new translation of the MMPI for Puerto Rican adolescents which revealed that both clinical and normal groups evidenced profiles that were elevated compared to baseline norms. These findings are consistent with a summary of cross-cultural studies of the MMPI by Butcher and Clark (1979), which shows that elevated scores on the MMPI are common upon crossing language and cultural boundaries. Prewitt-Diaz et al. (1984) conclude that there is a strong need for the development of new norms indigenous to Puerto Rico.

The presence of differences between Hispanic norms and standardized white norms has been attributed by some critics to cultural bias in the MMPI. Because items are keyed to reflect psychopathology on an empirical basis, items indicative of pathology from standardization on Anglo-American diagnostic groups are not necessarily pathological, and are even common behaviors, feelings, and beliefs in different Hispanic subcultures (Padilla and Ruiz, 1975). For example, in Puerto Rican culture, it is common to practice spiritualism (Rogler and Hollingshead, 1985), an ideology that posits the existence of an invisible world of spirits (good or evil) who may penetrate the visible world to influence human lives, such as causing mental illness. When certain MMPI items (e.g., "Evil spirits possess me at times") are viewed in the context of spiritualistic traditions, certainly a pathological label cannot be automatically affixed to the Hispanic respondent.

Translation also poses a serious problem for cross-cultural researchers, particularly given the diversity of Hispanic subcultures (Gurak and Rogler, 1983). As Olmedo (1981) points out, there are lexical, morphological, syntactical, phonological, and idiomatic differences between languages. The problem of centricultural bias (Good and Good, 1986) refers precisely to the difficulties involved in translating a test developed in one culture into another culture's language. The content validity of the translation is questionable to the extent that behaviors considered pathological in the first culture are non-pathological in the other culture, and vice versa. The meaning of certain behaviors, as expressions of pathology, is not always preserved when crossing cultures—some culture-specific idioms do not have an adequate translation. The problem of adequacy of translation magnifies upon consideration of Hispanics' diversity. Differences exist between the Spanish spoken in Spain and that spoken in Latin America (cf. Olmedo, 1981), and similar differences exist in the Spanish spoken by Mexican-Americans, Puerto Ricans, and Cubans (Padilla and Ruiz, 1973). The implications of the translation problem for psychological test development are staggering. If we adhere strictly to the primary APA standards recommended for testing practices (APA, 1985), should we require separate test forms, differing in item type and content, as well as separate norms for each distinct Hispanic subculture? There is little reason for optimism that such a goal could be achieved in the foreseeable future. The question is raised to stress that invalid assessment and consequently misdiagnosis of Hispanics loom as real possibilities if our psychometric technology does not satisfy primary standards for personality testing.

The question of potential bias in psychological tests has not been exclusively defined by comparisons of normative distributions of test scores between different ethnic groups. A somewhat more technical approach to test bias is to examine the internal or latent factor structure of tests across different populations. The internal structure of a test refers to the pattern of intercorrelation exhibited among the items composing the test in a given population. This implies not just a focus on whether the correlations among items are generally high or low (or positive or negative), which is a matter of internal consistency reliability, but also a focus on the subsets of items that cluster together as latent dimensions of the test. Factor analysis is the technique used to extract the latent dimensions or structure of tests, and the term factor invariance refers to the congruence of factor structures (or lack thereof) across different populations (e.g., Mulaik, 1971). Test bias is in evidence, therefore, if the factor structure of a given personality test differs between ethnic populations.

Although some attention has been given to assessing factor invariance by comparing different ethnic groups in the intelligence testing literature (e.g., Gutkin and Reynolds, 1981 a,b), there is little comparative factor analytic research on cross-cultural studies of personality tests—and even less research specific to Hispanic populations. Although it is not a personality inventory, the NIMH Center for Epidemiological Studies Depression Scale (CES-D) has been used as a screening device for depression, and it has been found to display similar factor structure among Anglo, black, and Mexican American groups (Aneshensel et al., 1983; Roberts, 1980). Thus, apart from other considerations of test bias, this scale can be presumed to be factorially invariant or unbiased in latent structure. Unfortunately, the CES-D does not provide a comprehensive personality profile, and it is used primarily in mental health or epidemiological research but not in clinical practice to facilitate diagnostic decision making.

Prewitt-Diaz et al. (1984) refer to "validity" in comparing the intercorrelations among MMPI scales on a Spanish translation of the MMPI with the intercorrelations in the norm group. Their finding that the pattern of MMPI scale correlations is congruent between the Spanish translation and the standard English version is more appropriately considered as evidence tangential to factor invariance—similar patterns of intercorrelations imply similar factor structures. In a study of the MMPI administered in English to groups of white, black, and Mexican American prison inmates, Holland (1979) reported differences in both the number of MMPI dimensions and the composition of those dimensions as a function of ethnicity. Within the white inmate group, three factors emerged which corresponded to the factor structure reported in earlier MMPI research. However, within the black and Mexican American groups, four factors emerged which were dissimilar between the two minority groups and which also bore little resemblance to the three white factors. Holland was unable to provide a substantive interpretation of the nature of the dimensions extracted in the black and Mexican American groups, and cautioned that the reference to white norms with black and Mexican American examinees could result in misleading diagnoses. Holland is in agreement with Gynther's (1972) earlier recommendation of separate norms for different ethnic groups, and he forecasts that the questionable practice of interpreting minority group members' MMPI profiles in terms of white standards is likely to persist ". . . along with the erroneous conclusions it produces, until further information becomes available about the distinctive characteristics of MMPI performance among these groups" (p.72).

In anticipation that factor analytic studies of the MMPI and other personality tests will eventually be conducted in different cultural contexts, as might be expected from the growing body of cross-cultural MMPI literature, we can only hope that they will be done properly. Olmedo (1981) notes that there are technical psychometric problems in determining the congruence of factors across populations, and he recommends confirmatory factor analytic techniques to determine how well the factor structure extracted in one population fits the factor structure in another population. Mulaik (1972) provides perhaps the most comprehensive discussion of the problem and maps out the assumptions and procedures necessary to establish factor invariance across populations. The problem of establishing factor invariance is clearly a serious one for personality tests with a multidimensional personality profile since, as we have seen, the same dimensions may not underlie the observed profiles of Anglo and Hispanic examinees. Factor invariance seemingly would not be a source of bias in tests of unidimensional personality constructs—provided that unidimensionality and item analysis are confirmed across cultures and Spanish-language translations.

Two other popular definitions of test bias refer to differential validity and differential prediction. The concern for differential validity takes the form of a question about the equivalence across populations of the correlation between a test and an external criterion (e.g., Cole, 1981). Differential prediction, on the other hand, is a question of the equivalence across populations of external criterion scores predicted by the same test score (e.g., Drasgow, 1982). The two concerns are not redundant. A test can demonstrate comparable validity across populations in the sense that the magnitude of correlation coefficients is not significantly different, yet application of diverse regression equations can yield very different predicted criterion scores for members of different populations with the same test score. Conversely, a test may yield the same predicted score for members of different populations—if the regression equations are the same—but predictions in one population may be more accurate than predictions in another (since the correlations are significantly different).

The personality testing literature also reveals a general neglect of concern for differential validity and prediction with Hispanic populations. Although some attempts have been made to ensure comparable reliability (internal consistency and test-retest) estimates of Spanish translations of personality tests (e.g., Lubin et al., 1986; Prewitt-Diaz et al., 1984; Argulewicz and Miller, 1984), predictive validity has rarely been investigated, and differential validity and prediction involving direct comparisons of correlation coefficients and regression equations does not appear in the literature. Nevertheless, there are issues in the mainstream of the psychometric literature on test bias which will be instructive to researchers studying differential validity and prediction in Hispanic populations.

A more fundamental question of test bias concerns the concept of "measurement equivalence," which refers to the relationship between observed test scores and underlying latent abilities or traits across different populations (Drasgow, 1982, 1984). Test bias in terms of measurement nonequivalence is evident when the relationship between test scores and the latent trait (i.e., personality characteristic) varies across populations; that is, examinees of different ethnic groups with the same latent personality trait value achieve different observed personality test scores. There is no necessary assumption that either the latent trait or observed test scores must have different means across groups, or for the test scores to differentially correlate with or differentially predict an external criterion in order for the test to be considered biased according to the definition of measurement equivalence. Rather, test bias at this most fundamental level indicates that observed test scores take on a different meaning within different ethnic groups.

Drasgow (1982) reviewed the literature on test bias—which is focused on ability and aptitude testing, not personality testing—in light of the common finding that there is little evidence of bias reported for most tests, based on statistical evaluations of differential validity. He provided examples of simulated test bias in one examinee group but not in another of equal ability and showed that under the condition of measurement non-equivalence, statistical tests are insensitive to differential validity. Since statistical tests are virtually incapable of detecting differential validity when measurement equivalence is not satisfied, the vast majority of differential validity studies conducted to date are meaningless. Therefore, Drasgow concluded that they "cannot be used as evidence that tests are 'fair' to ethnic and cultural minority groups" (1984, p. 135). Thus, when validity studies of personality tests are eventually conducted, we support Drasgow's recommendation that measurement equivalence is a prerequisite condition which must be established prior to evaluation of a test's differential validity. Procedures for establishing measurement equivalence are discussed in Lord (1980).

Turning to the literature on projective personality testing we find that Hispanic and black examinees consistently have been evaluated as less verbally fluent, less emotionally responsive, and more psychopathological than their non-minority counterparts (Ames and August, 1966; Booth, 1960; Costantino and Malgady, 1983). These findings raise questions as to whether minority children are inherently deficient in verbal skills and predisposed to psychological disorder or, again, whether traditional projective techniques fail to accurately measure the personality functioning of linguistic and cultural minority children. The latter hypothesis presents a compelling problem which is more basic than issues of criterion-related validity of projective tests inasmuch as it is widely acknowledged that content scores (e.g., achievement motivation) of inarticulate examinees are invalidated by examinees' lack of verbal fluency (e.g., McClelland, 1953; Smith, 1970). To the extent that projective test stimuli, such as the ambiguous non-minority figures of the Thematic Apperception Test (TAT), are not congruent with the cultural experiences of examinees, lack of identification with the characters, symbols and setting in the stimuli may inhibit verbal fluency and hence preclude a valid clinical assessment of personality functioning (cf. Anderson and Anderson, 1955). Apart from the usual psychometric reservations about low reliability and validity which are often voiced about projective techniques even with non-minority examinees (e.g., Anastasi, 1981), it is difficult to understand why such assessment practices prevail with ethnic and linguistic minority examinees when it is known that the validity of projective tests is impugned with inarticulate examinees.

Early attempts to modify the standard TAT for black examinees generated mixed outcomes, some studies reporting higher verbal fluency in response to black TAT figures (e.g., Bailey and Green, 1977; Cowan and Goldberg, 1967; Thompson, 1949) and others not (e.g., Korchin et al., 1950; Light, 1955; Schwarz et al., 1951). In the projective test literature with Hispanics, the TEMAS (Tell-Me-A-Story) test (Costantino, 1987) has weathered psychometric scrutiny somewhat more favorably than efforts to create black TATs. The TEMAS test consists of colorful pictures of Hispanic and black characters interacting in urban settings. The pictures are less ambiguous than the usual projective test stimuli, and are structured to depict situations involving conflicting events (e.g., playing with friends vs. complying with a parental errand). The content of examinees' stories about the pictures can be objectively and reliably scored on a number of personality dimensions. The TEMAS profile consists of dimensions such as achievement motivation, aggression, depression, and reality testing, which provide for an integrated assessment leading to distinct diagnostic outcomes (Costantino et al., 1988). Psychometric research on the TEMAS test has demonstrated enhanced verbal fluency of Puerto Rican examinees in comparison to their stories on the TAT (Costantino et al., 1981; Costantino and Malgady, 1983); acceptable interrater and internal consistency reliability, and evidence of concurrent and predictive validity (Malgady et al., 1984); and clinical utility for discriminating between outpatients and non-clinical students functioning adaptively in school (Costantino et al., 1988). The TEMAS test has been standardized primarily with Puerto Rican children and adolescents in New York City, and with a limited sample of Cuban, Central and South American, and Mexican American children. Other cross-cultural studies of the TEMAS test have been conducted in San Juan, Puerto Rico, and in Buenos Aires, Argentina.

The developmental research conducted on the TEMAS test is probably the most intensive effort to standardize and validate a projective technique specific to a Hispanic population. Additional work on projective testing has been done in Spain by Espada (1986), who has undertaken the standardization and validation of the TAT with examinees ranging from 14 to 53 years old. Espada's efforts include the development of a comprehensive scoring system for the Spanish TAT, which accesses interpersonal relationships, aggression, depression, and achievement motivation. The developmental research on the TEMAS test and the Spanish TAT is consistent with the resurgence of interest in establishing objective scoring systems for projective techniques and the need to establish cross-cultural norms (Exner and Weiner, 1982; Dana, 1986).

The outcome of our discussion thus far points to a firm conclusion. The various technical psychometric definitions of test bias have been clearly articulated in the mainstream of literature on psychological testing. Test bias is evidenced by any one of the following conditions: differential normative performance, variance in factor structure, differential validity or prediction, or most fundamentally, measurement non-equivalence across ethnic or linguistic minority populations. The literature on personality testing of Hispanics has little to say about statistical confirmation of empirical test bias against Hispanics. Thus, defendants of current personality testing practices are correct in that there is little conclusive evidence confirming the need for separate norms or establishing differential psychometric properties of standardized personality tests in Hispanic populations. In turn, the most outspoken cries of test bias tend to be founded on issues of face validity, by summoning examples of test items or behavioral symptoms which are considered pathological in one culture but not in another. The underlying issue for the present is whether standardized personality tests should be presumed innocent of bias when crossing cultural and language barriers, or whether tests should be presumed guilty of bias until conclusive evidence is amassed which resolves the issue.

Since the substance of the arguments involved in the controversy involve statistical evidence, it is instructive to examine the logic of both positions in a statistical analogy. The traditional null hypothesis in statistical inference is that of "no difference," which is preserved until empirical evidence enables its rejection. Traditional statistical reasoning leads quite naturally to posing "no bias" as the null hypothesis in cross-cultural psychometric research; that is, the hypothesis which prevails either in the absence of contradictory evidence or until sufficient evidence is gathered to reject it. Thus, we are bound to retain the null hypothesis of no bias against Hispanics in the case of most personality tests, simply because no research has been conducted enabling a contradiction of the status quo. We assert that, in the absence of empirical evidence, the prevailing hypothesis should be "bias" as the status quo, since the consequences of being in error with this proposition would be less serious than with the "no bias" hypothesis. Of course, this speculation runs counter to the inductive nature of statistical logic in hypothesis testing and to the statistical methods suitable for testing propositions regarding the various definitions of test bias. However, similar thinking can be observed in the American Psychological Association's revised *Standards for Educational and Psychological Tests* (APA, 1985). The revised standards include numerous caveats against using norms, item content, and validity and prediction estimates with demographically, linguistically, and culturally different populations. Indeed, many of the new standards are designated as "primary," meaning that they should be satisfied for all tests.

The current state of our psychometric technology for cross-cultural research or clinical practice is especially distressing when evaluated against the 1985 *Standards,* which generally have not been satisfied in the personality literature. Although it is true that these standards are relatively recent, a decade has passed since the publication of rather incisive indictments of Hispanic testing practices (e.g., Padilla, 1979) and mental health services for Hispanic Americans in this country (Special Populations Sub-Task Panel on Mental Health of Hispanic Americans, 1978). The reverberations of the issue of test bias are felt in attempting to come to grips with the data on the mental health needs of Hispanic populations, as discussed in Phase One of the framework; in formulating policy and recommendations regarding mental health services for Hispanics; and in reconsidering the propriety of using standardized psychological tests in decision-making—diagnostic or otherwise—about Hispanic clients in clinical settings. It is to the latter setting that we now turn, to examine the influence of language and cultural factors on clinical judgment of psychopathology and diagnosis.

Ethnicity, Bilingualism, and Psychopathology

During the past two decades, clinicians and researchers alike have become increasingly aware of the potentially confounding influence of ethnicity and bilingualism on the expression and interpretation of psychopathology in psychiatric interviews. Psychiatric epidemiological reports of heightened rates of psychological disorder among ethnic minority clients have been attributed by some researchers to misdiagnosis on the basis of the notion that psychodiagnosis decreases in accuracy as the sociocultural distance between clinician and client increases (Gross et al., 1969). Adebimpe (1981) suggests that members of ethnic minority groups, in general, are at higher risk of misdiagnosis than mainstream majority patients. Reacting to the epidemiological literature reporting higher prevalence rates for Hispanics, Good and Good (1986) question whether such studies reflect true differences in prevalence or "differences in judgments made by clinicians representing mainstream American culture or psychometric instruments that replicate such biases in judgment" (p. 5). They also cite research reexamining prevalence data (Hispanic inpatient diagnoses) by a research team of diagnosticians, the results of which suggest that as many as 75 percent of all Hispanic patients may be misdiagnosed. The implications of this statistic are staggering: to the extent that the effectiveness of psychotherapeutic intervention is predicated on accurate diagnosis, we would expect a similar rate of erroneous treatment decisions.

A number of reasons for the misdiagnosis of Hispanics have been offered. Karno (1966) observed that unacculturated Hispanics react to traditional non-minority clinicians with relative passivity, deference, and inhibited silence, thus leading clinicians to misinterpret the behavior they express in psychiatric interviews. Rogler and Hollingshead (1985) presented a portrayal and interpretation of an *ataque nervioso* (nervous attack) that may occur when a Hispanic person is confronted with an overwhelming stressful event. The nervous attack, which is characterized by screaming, falling, lack of communication, and agitated motor activity, was initially labeled the "Puerto Rican syndrome" by Veterans Administration psychiatrists who observed the disorder very frequently among Puerto Rican veterans. It is thought that the attack is a culturally patterned, acute hysterical reaction to an extremely stressful situation, but it is not a syndrome per se. However, if such an attack is not interpreted in its cultural context, an uninformed diagnostician may infer major pathology—mistakenly—from the collection of symptoms presented.

Good and Good (1986) identify three primary sources of bias in diagnosing ethnic minority clients: cultural differences associated with language (e.g., expression and meaning of symptoms, idioms of distress), institutionalized racism (e.g., cultural and racial stereotyping), and culturally based transference and countertransference (e.g., mode of relating to authority figures, denial of or over-identification with cultural values). They view these forms of bias as examples of a broader process which obtains from any diagnostic interaction—even without crossing cultural, linguistic, or socioeconomic boundaries. The diagnostician's own set of values and theoretical orientation prescribe an outlook that molds the evaluation of a patient's disclosures. Depending on a clinician's values and orientation, a wide degree of latitude is induced into the diagnosis rendered about a given patient. Similarly, Karno (1966) speculated that because the psychiatric "historical" interview derives from the medical model, an exclusionary bias operates in a manner which excludes sociocultural considerations from diagnosis (and later treatment planning) when in fact they may be crucial. The psychiatric interview focuses on the individual, not the individual's culture or the cultural context of the individual's problems.

Apart from clinicians' misinterpretation of their clients' self-disclosure of mental health problems, other evidence indicates that amount of self-disclosure is problematic in transactions between clinicians and patients of different ethnicity (e.g., Carkhuff and Pierce, 1967). Levine and Padilla's (1980) review of self-disclosure among Hispanic Americans, which is consistently reported to be less than that of Anglo Americans, has important implications for the diagnostic process because clinicians may find it difficult to obtain sufficient information of a personal and historical nature to formulate an accurate diagnosis.

Thus, for quite some time the research literature on psychiatric evaluation of Hispanics has alluded to the ubiquity of misdiagnosis by non-Hispanic clinicians, or insufficiency of patients' self-disclosure for diagnosis, presumably as a consequence of sociocultural barriers emerging in the clinician-patient interaction. Foremost among such barriers is the interplay between bilingualism and biculturalism (Karno and Edgerton, 1969). For example, Edgerton and Karno (1971) reported that English-dominant Hispanics were indistinguishable from non-Hispanics in responding to psychiatric vignettes, yet Spanish-dominant Hispanics tended to express cultural themes of fatalism, familism, and patriarchal authoritarianism, which often may be interpreted as pathological by non-Hispanic clinicians. The clinical implications of bilingualism and especially age at second-language acquisition were stressed by Peck (1974), who observed: first, that English acquisition in adulthood often leads to speech distortions, which in turn are misinterpreted due to clinicians' stereotypical attitudes toward bilinguals and, second, that bilinguals frequently experience a loss of second-language fluency under stressful conditions, such as in a psychiatric interview.

When the fact that bilingualism and language of interview are likely to influence the outcome of a psychiatric interview is acknowledged, the following questions arise: In which language, English or Spanish, do bilinguals express greater pathology? Which language conveys the true nature and extent of pathology? The literature focusing on the first question is equivocal, and the second question has still to be formally addressed.

On the basis of a small sample of clinical case histories, Del Castillo (1970) related from personal experience that Hispanic psychiatric patients appear highly psychotic when interviewed in Spanish but much less so when interviewed in English. From these observations Del Castillo reasoned that psychotic processes are ideationally represented in the native language but that the act of speaking a less familiar second language compels the patient into better reality contact. While this reasoning may indeed be correct, Del Castillo assumes that the language in which greater pathology is expressed necessarily conveys the true extent of pathology. Similar observations are offered by Ruiz (1975) and Gonzalez (1978), who reported that emotional responsiveness and intensity of pathology is greater in Spanish-language interviews. However, other studies have reached precisely the opposite conclusion.

Contrary to the findings of clinical observations, Marcos (1976) and his colleagues (Marcos et al., 1973 a, b) reported a series of experimental studies suggesting that English-speaking clinicians infer greater pathology during English interviews than do Spanish-speaking clinicians during Spanish interviews. Focusing on the dynamics of the psychiatric interview situation, Price and Cuellar (1981) and Vazquez (1982) later criticized the Marcos studies, independently recognizing significant sources of confounding in experimental design. Although Marcos carefully blinded his clinicians to the purpose of the study and minimized intrusive behavior on their parts, language of interview and ethnicity of the clinical diagnosticians were inextricably intertwined. Interestingly enough, when such confounding was eliminated—with bilingual Hispanic clinicians evaluating both English and Spanish interviews—the results contradicted Marcos' findings and corroborated Del Castillo's (1970) earlier observations of greater psychopathology being expressed in Spanish (Price and Cuellar, 1981).

Reacting to the confusion in the literature, Vazquez (1982) stressed the tentativeness of Del Castillo's case study approach and the inconclusiveness of Marcos' findings, which may be a function of interview language, sociocultural bias on the part of the clinicians, or both. Moreover, Vazquez proceeded to uncover sources of discrepancy between Marcos' studies and Price and Cuellar's modified replication. Whereas Marcos studied recent admissions to a large, urban psychiatric hospital, Price and Cuellar studied relatively chronic, hospitalized patients who were much more experienced in a psychiatric setting and who were treated in a culturally sensitive milieu. As Vazquez (1982) remarked, inexperienced patients indeed may express more pathology in English, but prior interviewing experience may promote greater self-disclosure and hence more apparent pathology in Spanish. Second, although bilingual clinicians evaluated both Spanish and English interviews, thus avoiding confounding of clinician ethnicity and language of interview, this paradoxically rendered tacit experimental blinding of the clinicians unlikely. Finally, Marcos eliminated possible intrusion of interviewer behavior on patient behavior through a standardized audiotaped interview, whereas Price and Cuellar attempted to preserve the ecological validity of the psychiatric interview with live interviews.

An earlier, related study by Hemphill (1971) also sheds some light on the language-of-interview controversy. Hemphill cited case histories of "true" polyglots (equally proficient in two languages), who reported auditory hallucinations only in their native language, and "refugee" polyglots (less proficient in their secondary language), who reported hallucinations only in their second language and explicitly denied the hallucinations in their native language. Hence it may be that failure to consider language dominance is an additional source of confounding between studies of psychiatric interviews of Hispanic patients. Perhaps Spanish-dominant bilinguals express greater pathology in English interviews, and coordinate or balanced bilinguals express greater pathology in Spanish interviews. As Lopez (in press) has recently commented, both groups of studies may present a glimpse of the truth—what is needed is an understanding of the complexity of patient and therapist interactions leading to differential judgments of pathology with bilingual patients. Clearly, the dynamic interplay of sociocultural and linguistic factors in the psychiatric interview needs to be experimentally disentangled in future programmatic research efforts. Only by this means can an understanding be achieved of the true nature and extent of psychopathology experienced by bilingual Hispanic patients, and the conditions under which clinicians arrive at discordant judgments of their psychopathology.

The literature on the language-of-interview controversy has been largely atheoretical; the ad hoc, empirical nature of this controversy has precluded a synthesis of discrepant research findings. Needed in addition to sound experimental design are carefully deduced hypotheses—drawn from the theoretical literature on the relationship between language and thought processes—enabling the testing of logically derived propositions rather than casual observations in an ad hoc fashion. Such research must also confront questions about which language, English or Spanish, expresses true pathology and whether there are discernible qualitative differences in clinical judgments as a function of bilingualism (e.g., what is the DSM-III concordance between English and Spanish interviews?) Even if the language-of-interview controversy is resolved, in the absence of a solid theoretical foundation one cannot assume that the language of more pathology is also the language of true pathology. Likewise, if the language of more pathology and true pathology are discovered, one cannot assume that misdiagnosis will be more likely in the less expressive or less appropriate language.

Before ending this chapter, we divert for a moment from issues of research to address the clinician troubled by the lack of attention given to cultural nuances in standard diagnostic criteria, such as the DSM-III (Lopez and Nuñez, 1987). As Lopez and Hernandez (1987) observe, clinicians have few empirically based guidelines for how to take culture into account in rendering diagnoses, and are "apt to develop their own notions of how and when culture should be considered" (p. 125). Thus, well-intentioned clinicians may be applying inappropriate cultural considerations to their Hispanic patients, who may vary dramatically in language proficiency, acculturation, and socioeconomic status. Good and Good

(1986) take this issue even further by recommending that a cultural axis be developed and added to the DSM-III. The axis would incorporate "emic" perceptions of the psychological problem by taking into account the viewpoint of the client and his/her primary social groups.

In bringing these issues to the attention of clinicians working with Hispanic clients, an initial tactic is to stress a list of sociocultural dimensions on which Anglo Americans and Hispanic Americans characteristically differ (e.g., Rosado, 1980; Sue, 1981). For example, unlike Anglo Americans, Hispanic Americans often display a greater concern for immediacy and the "here and now," as opposed to a more futuristic orientation in Anglo American culture; an external locus of control, causality being attributed to factors such as luck, supernatural powers, and God; an extended family support system, rather than a nuclear family; a concrete tangible approach to life, rather than an abstract, long-term outlook; a unilateral communication pattern with authority figures, such as avoidance of eye contact, deference, and silence as signs of respect; and multilingual language behavior, ranging from English to Spanish, to "Spanglish," a hybrid of the two. Although non-Hispanic clinicians ought to bear such Hispanic "traits" in mind when conducting an interview or interpreting test responses, taken too literally, broad generalizations about another culture easily invite stereotyping.

With a general idea of Hispanic characteristics taken into account, however, the clinician is in a position to approach the problem of assessment and diagnosis in a more informed, individualized manner, considering the client's particular Hispanic subculture, linguistic skills, and degree of acculturation. Ruiz (1981) reminds us that Hispanics can range in acculturation from "completely Hispanic" to "completely Anglo" but that most fall somewhere in between these extremes. Some Hispanic Americans who are acculturated may feel themselves more a part of Anglo American society, whereas others may reject it entirely, and still others may retain a bicultural identity. It is also not uncommon for acculturation to be situation-specific or compartmentalized in the sense that one may act Anglo American and speak English at work, for example, but maintain a traditional Hispanic lifestyle and speak Spanish at home.

What becomes abundantly clear from this discussion is that prior to administering a standard assessment battery or even a probing psychiatric interview, the diagnostician must be aware of the client's linguistic and sociocultural background. At the least, this suggests a need for a preliminary assessment of the client's language dominance, proficiencies, and preference, as well as situation-specific assessment of the client's degree of identification with Anglo American versus Hispanic culture. The outcome of such a pre-assessment strategy might be that some Hispanic clients should be tested and interviewed in English and assigned a standard diagnosis. At the other extreme, the interview might be conducted entirely in Spanish, with standardized test data and diagnostic categories entirely abandoned. Without an individualized approach to consideration of culture in interpreting test data and assigning a diagnosis, the unsuspecting clinician can stray from the path of cultural sensitivity to stereotype.

Summary

The two research problems discussed in this chapter are intrinsically linked to the broader problem of how language and cultural variability perturb the process of mental health evaluation of Hispanics. At the apex of the problem is the dilemma of imposing culture-bound definitions of mental illness or psychiatric symptomatology on individuals from diverse ethnic and demographic backgrounds. Research needs to move beyond face validity arguments about lists of behaviors or symptoms which are characteristic of Hispanics, and are or are not pathological, to research which establishes a basis for defining mental health parameters in Hispanic subcultures. Such research not only will have sound scientific merit, but also may serve to divert attention from rhetorical to empirical debate.

Once empirically-based definitions of criteria for mental illness are established, research can effectively examine methods of evaluating mental health. Despite much concern about test bias and misdiagnosis in the psychiatric interview, research on methods of evaluating mental illness in Hispanics is scant, unsystematic, and steeped in experimental confusion. Future research needs to concentrate on those procedures which are most commonly employed in clinical practice, such as the MMPI, projective techniques, and the psychiatric interview. Questions of potential test bias and the empirical mystery of how language and culture influence the expression and interpretation of pathology in psychiatric interviews pave an inviting path for researchers in this phase of the framework.

References

Adebimpe, V.R. (1981). Overview: White norms and psychiatric diagnosis of black patients. *American Journal of Psychiatry* 138: 279-285.

American Psychological Association (1985). *Standards for Educational and Psychological Testing.* Washington, D.C.: Author.

Ames, L.M. and August, J. (1966). Rorschach responses of negro and white 5-to-10-year-olds. *Journal of Genetic Psychology* 109: 297-309.

Anastasi, A. (1981). *Psychological Testing.* New York: Macmillan.

Anderson, H. and Anderson, G. (1955). *An Introduction to Projective Techniques.* New York: Prentice-Hall.

Aneshensel, C.S., Clark, V.A. and Frerichs, R.R. (1983). Race, ethnicity and depression: A confirmatory analysis. *Journal of Personality and Social Behavior* 22: 385-398.

Argulewicz, E.N. and Miller, D.C. (1984). Self-report measures of anxiety: A cross-cultural investigation of bias. *Hispanic Journal of Behavioral Sciences* 6: 396-406.

Bailey, B.E. and Green, J. (1977). Black thematic apperception test stimulus material. *Journal of Personality Assessment* 41: 25-30.

Booth, L.J. (1960). A normative comparison of the responses of Latin American and Anglo American children to the children's apperception test. In M.R. Haworth (Ed.), *The C.A.T.: Facts about Fantasy.* New York: Grune and Stratton.

Butcher, J.N. and Clark, L.A. (1979). Recent trends in cross-cultural MMPI research and application. In J.N. Butcher (Ed.), *New Developments in the Use of the MMPI* (pp. 69-112). Minneapolis: University of Minnesota Press.

Carkhuff, R. and Pierce, R. (1967). Differential effects of therapist race and social class upon depth of self-exploration in the initial clinical interview. *Journal of Consulting Psychology* 31: 632-634.

Cole, N.S. (1982). Bias in testing. *American Psychologist* 36: 1067-1077.

Costantino, G. (1987). *The TEMAS Test* (Minority Version). Los Angeles: Western Psychological Services.

Costantino, G. and Malgady, R.G. (1983). Verbal fluency of Hispanic, black and white children on TAT and TEMAS, a new thematic apperception test. *Hispanic Journal of Behavioral Sciences* 5: 199-206.

Costantino, G., Malgady, R.G. and Vazquez, C. (1981). A comparison of Murray's TAT and a new thematic apperception test for urban Hispanic children. *Hispanic Journal of Behavioral Sciences* 3: 291-300.

Costantino, G., Malgady, R.G. and Rogler, L.H. (1988). *Technical Manual: The TEMAS Test.* Los Angeles: Western Psychological Services.

Costantino, G., Malgady, R.G., Rogler, L.H. and Tsui, E. (1988). Discriminant analysis of clinical outpatients and public school children by TEMAS: A thematic apperception test for Hispanics and blacks. *Journal of Personality Assessment* 52: 670-678.

Cowan, G. and Goldberg, E. (1967). Need achievement as a function of the race and sex of figures of selected TAT cards. *Journal of Personality and Social Psychology* 5: 245-249.

Dana, R.H. (1986). Thematic apperception test used with adolescents. In A.I. Rabin (Ed.), *Projective Techniques for Adolescents and Children* (pp.14-36). New York: Springer.

Del Castillo, J. (1970). The influence of language upon symptomatology in foreign-born patients. *American Journal of Psychiatry* 127: 242-244.

Drasgow, F. (1982). Biased test items and differential validity. *Psychological Bulletin* 92: 526-531.

Drasgow, F. (1984). Scrutinizing psychological tests: Measurement equivalence and equivalent relations with external variables are the central issues. *Psychological Bulletin* 95: 134-135.

Echevarria, C., De la Torre, J., Garcia Santa-Cruz, Y. and Africa, M. (1969). Relación entre actitudes interpersonales, neuroticismo y rasgos psicopáticos en universitarios españoles (MMPI y SIV). *Revista de Psicologia General y Aplicada* 24: 894-901.

Edgerton, R. B. and Karno, M. (1971). Mexican-American bilingualism and the perception of mental illness. *Archives of General Psychiatry* 24: 286-290.

Espada, A.A. (1986). *Manual Operativo para el Test de Apercepción Temática.* Madrid, Spain: Ediciones Piramide.

Exner, J.E. and Weiner, I.B. (1982). *The Rorschach: A Comprehensive System. Assessment of Children and Adolescents* (vol.3), New York: Wiley and Sons.

Fuller, C.G. and Malony, N.H. (1984). A comparison of English and Spanish (Nuñez) translations of the MMPI. *Journal of Personality Assessment* 48: 130-131.

Garcia, J. (1977). Intelligence testing: Quotients, quotas, and quackery. In

J.L. Martinez (Ed.), *Chicano Psychology* (pp. 197-212). New York: Academic Press.

Gonzalez, J.R. (1978). Language factors affecting treatment of bilingual schizophrenics. *Psychiatric Annals* 8: 68-70.

Good, B.J. and Good, M.J. (1986). The cultural context of diagnosis and therapy: A view from medical anthropology. In M.R. Miranda and H.H. Kitano (Eds.), *Mental Health Research and Practice in Minority Communities: Development of Culturally Sensitive Training Programs* (pp. 1-27). Washington, D.C.: National Institute of Mental Health, Minority Research Resources Branch, Division of Biometry and Applied Sciences.

Gross, H., Knatterud, G. and Donner, L. (1969). The effect of race and sex on the variation of diagnosis and disposition in a psychiatric emergency room. *Journal of Nervous and Mental Diseases* 148: 638-642.

Gurak, D.T. and Rogler, L.H. (1983). Hispanic migrants in New York settlement. Renewal application submitted to the Department of Health and Human Services, Washington, D.C.

Gutkin, T.B. and Reynolds, C.R. (1981 a). Factorial similarity of the WISC-R for Anglos and Chicanos referred for psychological services. *Journal of School Psychology* 18: 34-39.

Gutkin, T.B. and Reynolds, C.R. (1981 b). Factorial similarity of the WISC-R for white and black children from the standardization sample. *Journal of Educational Psychology* 73: 227-231.

Gynther, M.D. (1972). White norms and black MMPIs: A prescription for discrimination? *Psychological Bulletin* 78: 386-402.

Gynther, M.D. and Green, S.B. (1980). Accuracy may make a difference, but does a difference make for accuracy? A response to Pritchard and Rosenblatt. *Journal of Consulting and Clinical Psychology* 48: 268-272.

Hemphill, R.E. (1971). Auditory hallucinations in polyglots. *South African Medical Journal* 45: 1391-1394.

Holland, T.R. (1979). Ethnic group differences in MMPI profile pattern and factorial structure among adult offenders. *Journal of Personality Assessment* 43: 72-77.

Karno, M. (1966). The enigma of ethnicity in a psychiatric clinic. *Archives of General Psychiatry* 14: 516-520.

Karno, M. and Edgerton, R.B. (1969). Perception of mental illness in a Mexican community. *Archives of General Psychiatry* 20: 233-238.

Korchin, S.J., Mitchell, H.E. and Meltzoff, J. (1950). A critical evaluation of the Thompson Thematic Apperception Test. *Journal of Projective Techniques* 14: 445-452.

Levine, E.S. and Padilla, A.M. (1980). *Crossing Cultures in Therapy: Pluralistic Counseling for the Hispanic.* Monterey, California: Brooks/Cole Publishing.

Light, B.H. (1955). A further test of the Thompson TAT rationale. *Journal of Abnormal Social Psychology* 51: 148-150.

Lopez, S. (in press). Empirical basis of ethnocultural and linguistic bias in mental health evaluations of Hispanics. *American Psychologist.*

Lopez, S. and Hernandez, P. (1987). When culture is considered in the evaluation and treatment of Hispanic patients. *Psychotherapy* 24: 120-126.

Lopez, S. and Nuñez, J.A. (1987). Cultural factors considered in selected diagnostic criteria and interview schedules. *Journal of Abnormal Psychology* 96: 270-272.

Lord, F.M. (1980). *Applications of Item Response Theory to Practical Testing Problems.* Hillsdale, N.J.: Erlbaum.

Lubin, B., Masten, W.G. and Rinck, C.M. (1986). Comparison of Mexican and Mexican American college students on the Spanish (American) version of the Depression Adjective Checklist. *Hispanic Journal of Behavioral Sciences* 8: 173-178.

Malgady, R.G., Costantino, G. and Rogler, L.H. (1984). Development of a thematic apperception test (TEMAS) for urban Hispanic children. *Journal of Consulting and Clinical Psychology* 52: 986-996.

Malgady, R.G., Rogler, L.H. and Costantino, G. (1987). Ethnocultural and linguistic bias in mental health evaluation of Hispanics. *American Psychologist* 42: 228-234.

Marcos, L.R. (1976). Bilinguals in psychotherapy: Language as an emotional barrier. *American Journal of Psychotherapy* 30: 552-560.

Marcos, L.R., Alpert, M., Urcuyo, L. and Kesselman, M. (1973a). The effect of interview language on the evaluation of psychopathology in Spanish-American schizophrenic patients. *American Journal of Psychiatry* 130: 549-553.

Marcos, L.R., Urcuyo, L., Kesselman, M. and Alpert, M. (1973b). The language barrier in evaluating Spanish-American patients. *Archives of General Psychiatry* 29: 655-659.

McClelland, D. (1953). *The Achievement Motive.* New York: Appleton-Century.

McClelland, D. (1973). Testing for competence rather than for "intelligence." *American Psychologist* 28: 1-14.

McCreary, C. and Padilla, E. (1977). MMPI differences among Black, Mexican-American, and White male offenders. *Journal of Clinical Psychology* 33: 171-177.

McGill, J.C. (1980). MMPI score differences among Anglo, black, and Mexican-American welfare recipients. *Journal of Clinical Psychology* 36: 147-151.

Mulaik, S. (1972). *The Foundations of Factor Analysis.* New York: McGraw-Hill.

Nuñez, R. (1967). *Inventario Multifásico de la Personalidad MMPI—Español.* Mexico City: El Manual Moderno.

Nuñez, R. (1968). *Aplicación del Inventario Multifásico de la Personalidad (MMPI) a la Psicopatología.* Mexico City: El Manual Moderno.

Olmedo, E.L. (1981). Testing linguistic minorities. *American Psychologist* 36: 1078-1085.

Padilla, A.M. (1979). Critical factors in the testing of Hispanic Americans: A review and some suggestions for the future. In R. Tyler and S. White (Eds.), *Testing, Teaching, and Learning: Report of a Conference on Testing* (pp. 219-243). Washington, D.C.: National Institute of Education.

Padilla, A.M. and Ruiz, R.A. (1973). *Latino Mental Health: A Review of the Literature* (DHEW Publication No. HSM 73-9143). Washington, D.C.: National Institute of Education.

Padilla, A.M. and Ruiz, R.A. (1975). Personality assessment and test interpretation of Mexican Americans: A critique. *Journal of Personality Assessment* 39: 103-109.

Page, R.D. and Bozlee, S. (1982). A cross-cultural MMPI comparison of alcoholics. *Psychological Reports* 50: 639-646.

Paz, J.M. (1952). La personalidad de los estudiantes de medicina, según el MMPI. Unpublished doctoral dissertation. University of Havana, Cuba.

Peck, E. (1974). The relationship of disease and other stress to second language. *International Journal of Social Psychiatry* 20: 128-133.

Prewitt-Diaz, J.O., Nogueras, J.A. and Draguns, J. (1984). MMPI (Spanish translation) in Puerto Rican adolescents: Preliminary data on reliability and validity. *Hispanic Journal of Behavioral Sciences* 6: 179-190.

Price, C. and Cuellar, I. (1981). Effects of language and related variables on the expression of psychopathology in Mexican American psychiatric patients. *Hispanic Journal of Behavioral Sciences* 3: 145-160.

Pritchard, D.A. and Rosenblatt, A. (1980). Reply to Gynther and Green. *Journal of Consulting and Clinical Psychology* 48: 273-274.

Reschly, D.J. (1981). Psychological testing in educational classification and placement. *American Psychologist* 36: 1094-1102.

Risetti, F. (1981). Clinical validity of the Chilean MMPI. Paper presented at the Seventh International Conference on Personality Assessment, Honolulu, Hawaii.

Roberts, R.E. (1980). Reliability of the CES-D scale in different ethnic contexts. *Psychiatry Research* 2: 125-134.

Rogler, L.H. and Hollingshead, A.B. (1985). *Trapped: Puerto Rican Families and Schizophrenia,* 3rd ed. Maplewood, N.J.: Waterfront Press.

Rosado, J.W. (1980). Important psychocultural factors in the delivery of mental health services to lower-class Puerto Rican clients: A review of recent studies. *Journal of Community Psychology* 8: 215-226.

Ruiz, E.J. (1975). Influence of bilingualism on communication in groups. *International Journal of Group Psychotherapy* 25: 391-395.

Ruiz, R.A. (1981). Cultural and historical perspectives in counseling Hispanics. In D.W. Sue (Ed.), *Counseling the Culturally Different: Theory and Practice* (pp. 186-215). New York: Wiley and Sons.

Schwartz, E., Riess, B. and Cottingham, A. (1951). Further critical evaluation of the negro version of the TAT. *Journal of Projective Techniques* 15: 394-400.

Smith, J. (1970). A note on achievement motivation and verbal influence. *Journal of Projective Techniques and Personality Assessment* 34: 121-124.

Special Populations Sub-Task Panel on Mental Health of Hispanic Americans (1978). *Report to the President's Commission on Mental Health.* Los Angeles: Spanish-Speaking Mental Health Research Center, University of California at Los Angeles.

Sue, D.W. (Ed.) (1981). *Counseling the Culturally Different: Theory and Practice.* New York: Wiley and Sons.

Thompson, C.E. (1949). The Thompson modification of the thematic apperception test. *Journal of Projective Techniques* 12: 469-478.

Vazquez, C. (1982). Research on the psychiatric evaluation of the bilingual patient: A methodological critique. *Hispanic Journal of Behavioral Sciences* 4: 75-80.

Chapter 5

Phase Four: Psychotherapeutic Services

Mr. Pedro Rios needed to talk to someone about his feelings and problems. He felt he did not have a right to live because his mother told him she had tried to abort him. She explained that they were very poor and he would have been another mouth to feed. He thought of killing himself to relieve his suffering: everything was going to go wrong and something terrible was going to happen to his children. Sometimes his mind would go blank, or he felt so nervous he could neither sit nor lay down. Then he would walk aimlessly from one room to another, feeling sad. He could not talk to his relatives and friends about his feelings because they would think he was crazy. The therapist he had would not ask him questions because she wanted him to talk without being asked. But he could not express his feelings without being asked. The community mental health center he attended allowed him to change therapists. The new therapist asked him questions and he expressed his sadness. To improve his therapy, Mr. Rios brought to his new therapist two cassettes of tangos because it was important for her to understand the kind of music which fit his nostalgic feelings.

* * *

After the psychological evaluation of a patient, a treatment plan is developed based upon the patient's presenting symptoms and psychosocial history, the severity and diagnostic classification of the disorder, and the perceived prognosis of the patient. Phase Four of the conceptual framework begins when the treatment plan is implemented, either on an in- or outpatient basis, and ends when the patient leaves therapy, relieved of the psychological disorder or not.

Critics of mental health policies have echoed the theme that traditional psychotherapeutic services are both inappropriate and ineffective with Hispanic clients because they are not sensitive to Hispanic culture (e.g., Cohen, 1972; Costantino et al., 1986; Padilla et al., 1975; Rogler et al., 1987). These allegations are buttressed by the high attrition rates of Hispanics after initial therapeutic contact, and by claims of questionable therapeutic gains when

Hispanics continue in treatment. This chapter discusses two research problems related to the appropriateness and effectiveness of mental health treatment services that are provided to Hispanics.

The first research problem raises questions as to whether or not the content of culturally sensitive treatment modalities should bear an isomorphic, mirror-like relationship to the client's culture. This problem is exemplified by efforts in the literature to either select or modify traditional therapy modalities to be congruent with perceived features of Hispanic culture. The second research problem questions whether culturally sensitive therapy, in some circumstances, ought to depart from the isomorphic assumptions and redirect cultural elements to bridge the gap between the client's native culture and the majority culture. This problem is illustrated by treatment efforts which adapt Hispanic cultural features as a therapeutic vehicle to emphasize coping with the daily stresses of life in a host society with a different culture.

Our discussion of these two research problems differs somewhat from that in the previous chapters. This chapter moves away from the research literature, since there are very few studies which compare the effectiveness of different treatment interventions with Hispanics and non-Hispanics. Instead, we focus on the literature related to clinical practice and the effectiveness of attempts to render therapeutic modalities culturally sensitive. However, before discussing culturally sensitive psychotherapeutic methods, we briefly examine the issues giving impetus to these research problems: early attrition and ineffectiveness of traditional treatment modalities.

Whatever the mode of treatment used, the question of whether appointments will be kept and the treatment sustained is paramount. The literature widely acknowledges the fact that Hispanics have higher dropout rates than Anglo clients (e.g., Sue, 1981) Reasons for early attrition from therapy have included: low acculturation (Miranda, 1976); low socioeconomic status (Baekland and Lundwell, 1975); inability to perceive or label causal relationships between ideas and feelings pertinent to one's behavior (Baekland and Lundwell, 1975); and negative attitudes toward therapists and the benefits of therapy (Acosta et al., 1980). In fact, many of the ideas presented in Phase Two, seeking to explain patterns of utilization of mental health facilities, could be used to examine dropout rates among Hispanics, an issue which deserves the attention of research. This issue, however, is not examined in this chapter, which focuses on the relationship between culture and psychotherapeutic services.

The general question of whether or not therapy is more effective than no treatment has been much debated (e.g., Garfield, 1981). Since Eysenck's

(1952) early controversial claim that clients participating in therapy fared no better than those on a list waiting for therapy, his data have been re-analyzed and this claim disputed. The consensus of the profession seems to be that therapy is more effective than no treatment, as supported by reviews of the literature which classify studies according to which position they support (e.g., Luborsky et al., 1975). More recently, Smith and Glass' (1977) meta-analysis of psychotherapeutic outcome studies, which combined data from 375 studies, yielded the conclusion that the typical therapy client is better off than 75 percent of untreated clients.

The backbone of claims for culturally sensitive therapy for ethnic minority clients is Paul's (1967) general question: What type of psychotherapy administered by whom is most effective for which type of client with what type of problem under which set of circumstances? Consideration of the ethnic group of the client, the therapist, and the surrounding cultural ambiance adds a new perspective to these queries. Unfortunately, the studies which address therapy outcomes in the Hispanic population are small and incomplete fragments of the entire picture. In a recent examination of two decades of research on psychotherapeutic services for ethnic minorities in general, Sue (1988) identified two competing positions. The first is that ethnic or cultural differences between client and therapist decrease the probability of favorable therapeutic outcome. The second position, based on cross-cultural research on therapeutic outcomes, argues the opposite, viz., that cultural differences are irrelevant to therapeutic outcome.

Sue (1988) cites the extensive literature on racial and ethnic matching in psychotherapy, which primarily deals with blacks. Considering a number of studies which have failed to confirm ethnicity as a factor related to differential treatment outcomes, Sue provides a detailed list of methodological flaws which might explain this finding. He suggests that the problem of cultural differences in therapy has been misconceived. First of all, ethnicity should not be taken as a proxy for culture, as it has been in most studies. Ethnic differences embody a broader class of variables than culture, such as socioeconomic status, which confound interpretations of therapeutic effects attributed to culture. Second, based on an earlier argument (Sue and Zane, 1987), it may be unreasonable to expect strong effects of culture or ethnicity on therapeutic outcomes because they are distal or not directly linked to therapy gains. Sue and Zane suggest that consideration of culture or ethnicity in formulating treatment plans may enhance the process of therapy, which is proximally or more directly linked to therapeutic outcomes. An example of this would be evident if strong cultural similarities between client and therapist lead the client to perceive the therapist as having empathy, and this perception leads to a more favorable therapeutic out-come. Accordingly, Sue and Zane recommend that future research examine the role of culture in therapy by operationalizing the concept in terms of "concrete units," and then examine how such units are related to therapeu-tic processes and outcomes. The identity of such units, however, is left un-specified. The hypothesis that cultural effects are distal rather than proxi-mal to therapeutic outcome is worthy of being tested: it is important to uncover the extent to which cultural differences impact both directly and indirectly, as mediated by therapeutic process variables, on therapeutic out-comes.

Isomorphism and the Selection or Modification
of Treatments to Match Hispanic Culture

The first research problem derives from how the relationship between therapy and culture has been defined in the literature on culturally sensitive treatments for Hispanics. The prevailing definition emphasizes the point that therapy should bear a mirror-like relationship to Hispanic culture. The client's culture would form the basis for the selection or modification of the therapy. The isomorphic prescription appears reasonable because it is undergirded by the prevailing therapeutic norm that the client's culture should be respected, and that such respect increases the effectiveness of therapy. We shall treat these assertions as hypotheses forming part of the first research problem.

Before looking at specific examples of treatment modification in the inter-est of the client's culture, it is worth noting that individualized treatment is an alternative method of reaching the same goal of therapy. At the most specific and practical level of application, culturally sensitive therapy must accord with the needs of the individual client. In this context the work of Ruiz (1981) is a valuable addition to the elucidation of the concept of cultur-al sensitivity. Ruiz emphasizes the diversity of subcultures that fall under the catchall phrase "Hispanic," and the difficulty in identifying by surname a Hispanic, one who is bicultural, and one sufficiently assimilated to be con-sidered an Anglo. Ruiz advocates the assessment of a client's acculturation prior to therapy and the basing of treatment on objective assessment of the degree of biculturalism that the individual client manifests. He provides rich examples of the individualized treatment plans that could span the continu-um from the "most Hispanic" to the "most Anglo" client. Case material is presented to show that with the "most Hispanic" client what is needed is not psychodynamically oriented therapy but concrete help in dealing with

". . . realistic and irksome problems which daily confront people who are poor, undereducated, foreign looking . . ." (p. 203). With the "most Anglo" clients, the usual therapies could be used.

An example of how one might use this conception is further provided by Ruiz and Casas (1981) in their discussion of a counseling program for Chicano college students. The authors do not assume that all students identified as Chicano are necessarily candidates for a bicultural therapy program. Instead, they define the various forms of "marginality" and "biculturalism" in this population according to the degree of identification with both the minority and majority society. They then conclude that only those students whose commitment to their own culture is stronger than their commitment to the majority culture are appropriate candidates for culturally sensitive counseling.

Another example of this relativistic, individualized approach is provided by Gomez (1983) who developed a framework for the kind of cultural assessment that Ruiz advocates. Gomez used a "cultural assessment grid" to formulate a typology of four cultural/therapeutic dilemmas. The need for culturally sensitive treatment, then, is thought to depend on whether the cultural factors are part of the individual or of the environment and on whether they contribute to the problem or are resources that can help in solving it. Depending on the interaction of these dimensions, culturally sensitive treatment can mean different things for each individual client.

Some researchers and therapists have argued that decisions about treatment ought not to preclude the use of psychoanalytic concepts and techniques with ethnic minority clients. Maduro and Martinez (1974) present a cogent argument for the value of self-exploration among Mexican Americans, claiming that "more self-aware individuals are needed to confront insidious social realities in the outer world, as well as unconscious themes in the inner world" (p. 461). They believe that Jungian dream work is congruent to Mexican culture, since Mexican folkhealers often specialize in the interpretation of dreams, and that such traditional analytic treatments are accessible and appropriate to their Hispanic clientele.

Nonetheless, the attitudes of Maduro and Martinez represent a minority opinion. Mental health practitioners working in inner-city economically-depressed Hispanic neighborhoods were among the first to level criticism at insight-oriented psychoanalytic therapy as both uneconomical and irrelevant to the context of Hispanic life. Their widely shared image of the psychologically distressed Hispanic was of a person harrassed by problems of poverty, slum life, and lack of acculturation. The image of such a client, taking his or her place on the proverbial psychoanalytic couch for long-term therapy designed to nurture insight into repressed impulses, caricatured psychoanalysis as an absurdly inconsequential modality. For this reason, few psychoanalytic therapists sought to address Hispanics' emotional problems, and a pervasive view developed that insight-oriented techniques were too esoteric to respond to the massive stresses impinging upon the majority of Hispanic clients.

Other approaches to cultural sensitivity in psychotherapy have modified traditional treatment modalities in accordance with perceived features of Hispanic culture. Bluestone and Vela's (1982) work is an exception to the general belief about the ineffectiveness of insight-oriented therapy with Hispanics. They make proposals of how adjustments can be made in the use of insight-oriented therapy with Puerto Ricans living at the bottom of the New York City socioeconomic heap. They stress the following points: the therapist should emphasize the need for the patient to keep appointments on time; the therapist should explain that psychological problems are less clear-cut than medical problems, and that quick cures cannot be expected; the therapist should be authoritative without being authoritarian to avoid transference problems associated with Puerto Rican paternal authoritarianism; therapy should address the Puerto Rican client's tendency to maintain an oversolicitous attitude while acting out hidden aggressive feelings; the therapist should avoid encouraging the client's culturally patterned, passive dependency; the therapist should use humor, proverbs, and metaphors to lighten the therapeutic interaction in dealing with common thoughts and feelings; and the therapist should consider the client's culturally patterned difficulties in expressing aggressive feelings. Notwithstanding such adjustments, the authors still recognize that suitable candidates for insight-oriented intervention must be relatively free from external chaos, display a persistent motivation to remain in therapy and a long-term outlook on life, and have a capacity for insight. Bluestone and Vela make an important contribution in coming to grips with a difficult task which others have avoided. However, even with a liberal interpretation of these qualifications, traditional insight therapy would be an inappropriate modality for many, probably most, members of the high-risk New York City Puerto Rican population. Ruiz (1981) made the point bluntly, speaking in reference to treatment of inner-city Hispanic clients: "Do they need insights into the etiology of . . . paranoia? Do they need to become more introspective or psychodynamically oriented? The answer to these questions is negative" (p.202).

A clear example of using a specific and common element from the client's ethnic culture to complement and modify the provision of conventional therapy is Kreisman's (1975) account of treating two Mexican American female schizophrenics who thought themselves *embrujadas* (bewitched). Kreisman was operating within a traditional psychiatric hospital, in which psychotherapy and medication were the treatments offered. The relevance and importance of these treatments to the patients' cure were never questioned by ward personnel. The essence of Kreisman's treatment modification was only to concur with the women that they were indeed bewitched. Encouraging the patients to perform their rituals and take the folk herbs in addition to traditional medications was enough to enable the establishment of a therapeutic rapport which persisted throughout treatment, the topic of folk illness subsequently ceasing to be an issue. Thus the therapists' acknowledgement of bewitchment and of the need for the techniques of the folk healer broke through the plateau which the conventional therapy had reached, and enabled further therapeutic progress to occur.

Reflecting on this experience, Kreisman formulates three alternative responses to a patient's cultural conception of the illness: it may be ignored; accepted as an equal but separate treatment; or encouraged and integrated into the treatment under the control of the therapist. Kreisman advocates the third approach; interestingly, he does not formulate the alternative of abandoning conventional treatment and developing a folk-healing therapy specific to these patients' needs. This approach might indeed be impossible within an inpatient psychiatric setting, although theoretically such an orientation would be basic to some alternative forms of cultural sensitivity. In the context of Kreisman's study, the display of cultural sensitivity in treatment means the clear and direct incorporation of elements from the patient's cultural patterns into the therapists' techniques without abandoning or compromising in any way the therapists' own conceptions and purpose.

A somewhat different example of using an element of the client's culture to modify traditional therapy is provided by the language-switching techniques employed by Pitta et al. (1978), who note a therapeutic potential within the bilingualism that characterizes most Hispanic clients. They postulate that emotional expression is freer and more spontaneous in one's native tongue, whereas the use of a second language fosters intellectual defenses and control. The language in which therapy is conducted is chosen according to both patient characteristics and phase of treatment, and language-switching is used as a therapeutic technique. The medium into which this technique is incorporated is a traditional, insight-oriented psychotherapy which is in no way modified for the needs of the ethnic client. Like Kreisman, these authors do not change their conception of therapy or the therapeutic role, but only utilize a perceived characteristic of their patient population in order to buttress and strengthen their chosen therapeutic medium.

Another way that culturally sensitive treatment can be implemented is through the enactment of culturally familiar roles during therapy, as shown by Maldonado-Sierra and Trent's (1960) early work with Puerto Rican schizophrenic patients. They used a three-member therapeutic team which was designed to reproduce what they assumed to be the typical Puerto Rican family structure. A senior psychiatrist played the role of the authoritative, dominant, aloof father; a mature psychiatric social worker, the role of the submissive, nurturant, martyr-like mother; and a psychiatric resident, the role of the older sibling who functions as a bridge connecting the other siblings, i.e., the schizophrenic patients to the surrogate parents. As an older sibling, the psychiatric resident develops brotherly familiarity with the schizophrenic patients and thus is able in group sessions to express the repressed hostilities of the "children" (patients) toward authority figures. This familial reenactment is thought to speed the therapeutic process by side-stepping the deep and repressed hostility of Puerto Rican patients to authority figures, which is thought to be a major reason for therapeutic resistance.

Thus, Maldonado-Sierra and Trent have taken a perceived characteristic of Hispanic patients and employed it in order to facilitate a traditional form of therapeutic intervention, i.e., inpatient group psychotherapy. The cultural characteristic here is a generalized model of the Puerto Rican family, one which disregards social class and regional variations on the island. Unlike Kreisman and Pitta et al., the authors do not use a cultural characteristic that the patients have already introduced into the treatment but instead impose their own perceptions of Puerto Rican culture onto the client, thus risking the possibility of stereotyped misjudgement. It is to avoid just such forms of stereotyping that authors such as Ruiz (1981) and Gomez (1983) advocate individualized assessment of cultural status and traits. Clearly, there are both benefits and risks to the utilization of perceived cultural traits in the adaptation and facilitation of established therapeutic modalities.

These studies of treatment selection or modification have employed individualized therapy, family therapy, and insight-oriented therapy as treatment modalities to increase the congruence between the therapeutic milieu and their Hispanic clientele. Such efforts are contributions to the clinical literature; however, the root research problem here is that the utility of treatment selections or modifications needs to be evaluated in carefully designed therapy outcome studies. Simply put, the research has not been conducted. Similarly, we cannot assume that culturally sensitive treatment decisions are always effective. This observation is crucial in encouraging future therapeutic outcome studies when we recall Sue and Zane's (1987) hypothesis that considerations of culture in therapy may be only distally related to concrete therapeutic outcomes.

The examples provided so far designate limited or small-scale adaptations of therapy based on aspects of the Hispanic client's culture which have been noted by clinicians in the field but have not been evaluated by research. A broader organizational adaptation, which has undergone scrutiny for therapeutic effectiveness, is "Unitas," a therapeutic community in the South Bronx of New York City serving primarily Puerto Rican youngsters (Farber and Rogler, 1981). About half of the Unitas participants are referred to the program by parents or teachers as problem children, usually because of withdrawn or bizarre behavior.

In order to counteract the stressful effects of single-parent households and family disorganization prevalent in the area, Unitas has created a system of symbolic families, each composed of up to 15 boys and girls usually living in the same neighborhood. Each symbolic family is headed by one or two older neighborhood teenagers who play the roles of symbolic mother, father, aunts, and uncles. These teenagers receive intensive training in psychological therapy and clinical skills and become the primary caretakers and therapists of the younger children, assuming many of the roles and functions that the children's real families have abdicated or lost.

An evaluation of Unitas was conducted by comparing a group of six-week summer participants with a comparable group of participants in a Police Athletic League (PAL) summer program (Procidano and Glenwick, 1985). It was found that Unitas participants increased significantly more in satisfaction with social support than the PAL participants, although most of the summer activities of the two programs were similar. Therefore, the enhancement of feelings of social support appear to be attributable to the therapeutic nature of the program and its symbolic family structure. It was also found that many participants in the Unitas program were self-referred and that those of the lowest socioeconomic status persisted longest in the program. Viewed in terms of the consistent finding that lower socioeconomic status is associated with early termination of therapy, the Unitas program seems to have a unique distinction—the most marginated children in the community are not only self-referring, but also remain longer in the program.

Unitas is an integrated treatment program which responds to the perceived needs of the lowest socioeconomic class into which many Puerto Rican clients fall. Although most of the features addressed characterize impoverished families generally, other patterns are recognized as aspects of the families' ethnicity. For example, Puerto Ricans differ from blacks in confronting myriad problems stemming from their unacculturated status and the troublesome disparities they experience between their values and language and those of the host society. Whereas inner-city Puerto Ricans and blacks share many characteristics, such as a family structure that is increasingly based on a single parent and in which siblings operate as the primary socializing agent, there are many crucial distinctions. Minuchin and his collaborators (1967), who have developed therapeutic interventions to address the problems of disorganized slum families, stress the strong cultural traditions which bolster Puerto Rican family roles and the dynamics of the Anglo-Hispanic culture clash that many Puerto Rican families experience. In the discussion of cultural sensitivity, therefore, it is important to distinguish between treatment adjustments made in the interest of socioeconomic-related factors as distinct from ethnically based cultural factors; otherwise, the targets of therapy can easily become blurred.

In the evaluation of future programmatic efforts such as Unitas, once again, Sue and Zane (1987) would remind us of the importance of disentangling the specific effects of cultural factors on outcomes. Although the results of the evaluation of Unitas are encouraging—particularly since any evaluative data represent a welcome addition to the literature—global treatment evaluations tell us little about the specific therapeutic processes associated with beneficial treatment outcomes. On the other hand, global evaluations are useful to practitioners interested in replicating entire treatment programs in other settings.

One of the most ambitious programmatic efforts made to adapt already existing treatment formats to the perceived needs of an Hispanic population is that of Szapocznik and his collaborators (1978). Their work begins with research that seeks to determine empirically the value orientations of Cubans and the ways in which such orientations differ from those of other racial and ethnic groups. They attempt to operationalize the concept of acculturation, which designates a problem widely experienced by Miami's Cubans as immigrants from a different sociocultural system. The concept and its measures form the basis of a theory of intrafamily tension and stress: the greater the disparity in acculturation between family members, the greater the family tensions and stresses. To treat the acculturative problems of Cuban families while being faithful to their cultural values and orientations, adaptations are introduced into ecological structural family therapy. This therapy integrates the approaches of ecological systems and structural family therapy, two available modalities, in order to ". . . permit the therapists to effect reorganization and restructuring by working with and utilizing the client's familial and extra-familial socioecological systems"

(Szapocznik et al., 1978, p. 113). The selection of family therapy is guided by the perceived familiocentric tradition of Cuban culture. At all times, the underlying premise is that treatment should ". . . respect and preserve the cultural characteristics of the Latin client" (p.113).

The point Szapocznik and his collaborators explicitly advance in their earlier research is that the treatment utilized should stand in an isomorphic, mirror-like relationship to the clients' cultural characteristics: ". . . the Cubans' value structure must be matched by a similar set of therapeutic assumptions" (Szapocznik et al., 1978, p. 116). The selection of family therapy as the treatment of choice is predicated on the notion that Cubans are family-oriented. Having determined through their research that the Cuban value system prized lineality, which is ". . . the preference for lineal relationships based on hierarchical or vertical structures . . ." (p.114), the family therapist assumes ". . . a position of authority within the family . . ." (p.119) in order to restore or reinforce parental authority over the children. Szapocznik and his colleagues outline a detailed sequence of therapeutic interventions, logically deduced from their empirical findings on the values of Cuban clients. Based on a deep respect for their clients' cultural heritage, this treatment replicates and reinforces essential elements of the Cuban value system and is, therefore, assumed to be culturally sensitive.

Of all the examples provided, it is Szapocznik's modification of family therapy to conform to Cuban values which most clearly expresses the assumption that cultural sensitivity is embodied in the isomorphic relationship between culture and therapy. However, this form of cultural sensitivity must still beckon research to test its effectiveness. It is essential that such research compare Hispanics with non-Hispanics, and culturally sensitive therapies with traditional (unmodified) therapies. If cultural sensitivity is indeed a worthwhile venture, Hispanics would be expected to demonstrate more favorable outcomes as the recipients of a culturally sensitive modality than as the recipients of an unmodified traditional modality; Hispanics would be expected to demonstrate less favorable outcomes than non-Hispanics as recipients of unmodified treatments; and these effects would be expected to be associated with the presence or absence of discrete units of cultural content in therapy. In such research, the criteria for assessing therapeutic outcomes must be multidimensional. In broader and more fundamental terms, the lowest common denominator is whether or not the client remains in therapy. If culturally sensitive treatment selections and modifications reduce attrition more than unmodified traditional treatments, this itself provides some justification for their use. It would be instructive also to assess the participants' and therapists' perceptions of the benefits of therapy and attitudes toward each other and the therapeutic process. If cultural sensitivity in therapy leads to greater client and therapist satisfaction, this too would support the use of such techniques in clinical practice. Finally, the most convincing evidence of the efficacy of cultural sensitivity would be research which unequivocally links cultural content in therapy to the remediation of the Hispanic client's emotional or behavioral disorder.

Departure from the Isomorphic Assumption in the
Development of New Treatments

The second research problem departs from the first problem by raising a question as to whether or not treatment modifications in the interest of cultural sensitivity ought to invariably preserve the culture isomorphically in therapy. More recently, Szapocznik et al. (1980) acknowledged that some treatment modifications with Hispanic clients need not follow an isomorphic pattern with respect to culture. Sometimes the objective of treatment is to change culturally prescribed behavior. For example, Boulette (1976) notes the frequency of the "subassertiveness" behavioral pattern in Mexican American women and judges this pattern to be psychologically dysfunctional. Research has demonstrated that this general sex-role pattern prevails in other Hispanic groups; for example, among Puerto Rican women of humble social-class origins it is a reflection of culturally induced conformity and of the women's passive acceptance of their lot in life (Rogler and Hollingshead, 1985). Boulette has targeted this culturally prevalent pattern as the focus of a therapeutic program that trains Mexican American women to be more assertive. The ultimate purpose of this training is for the women to overcome the somatic complaints, depression, and anxiety that are thought to result from culturally prescribed submissiveness.

The juxtaposition of the earlier assumptions of Szapocznik and his collaborators with those of Boulette raises critical questions: Once the cultural characteristics of a minority ethnic group have been adequately documented and researched, how should the characteristics be taken into account during treatment? Is effective therapy necessarily that which attempts the preservation of traditional cultural elements, or should acculturation, assimilation, or adaptation to the surrounding society sometimes take priority? Perhaps advocacy on behalf of preserving traditional cultural elements, no matter how well intentioned, ought not always or exclusively shape the character of therapeutic interventions. On the other hand, the values of the host society should similarly not be idealized as reflecting universal standards of mental health. It is our contention that when therapies are modified to address the needs of Hispanic clients, the adapted therapy need not isomorphically reflect the client's cultural characteristic. We hypothesize, therefore, that therapeutic gains can sometimes be made when traditional cultural patterns are bent, changed, or redirected according to predetermined therapeutic goals.

Thus, the first step in any process of treatment modification is to acknowledge or determine through research the special cultural characteristics that exist within a group; this recognition is then transformed into culturally sensitive programs. The kind of innovation that emerges depends, however, not only on the ethnic characteristics identified, but also on the therapeutic goals. Isomorphic reinforcement of cultural traits implies a deep respect for the cultural context, an underlying conservative cultural ideology, and an assumption that culturally transmitted elements are necessarily adaptive. Departures from such isomorphisms, on the other hand, assume that some cultural traits serve as an obstacle to cultural adaptation and that acculturation to the values of the host society is an additional and valid standard of adjustment. It also assumes that cultural elements can be modified within the treatment according to the implicit goals of the therapy without disputing their value and purpose as a culturally functional trait in the society of origin. It assumes, moreover, that research can be objective not only in terms of the assessment of Hispanic traits, but also in terms of the construction of culturally sensitive treatments.

The acceptance of this approach implies that culturally sensitive treatment can recognize and respect cultural values without isomorphically reflecting them in treatment. The therapeutic programs of Kreisman (1975), Maldonado-Sierra and Trent (1960), and Pitta et al. (1978) attempt to achieve cultural sensitivity by adhering to traditional treatment methods, with the cultural adaptations appended in order to facilitate the traditional treatment format. Although there are clear benefits to maintaining established therapeutic conceptions, the question still remains as to whether or not non-isomorphic cultural sensitivity can be incorporated into the development of innovative, culturally-specific treatment modalities.

To our knowledge there is only one study in the literature focusing upon this research problem which compares therapeutic outcomes of isomorphic and non-isomorphic culturally sensitive modalities. For this reason the study will be discussed in some detail. Costantino et al. (1986) report on the development of *cuento* or folktale therapy, as a form of behavior modeling therapy, for Puerto Rican children. The therapy takes as its medium the folktales of Puerto Rican culture, and as the premise of the therapeutic intervention, the importance of the transmission of such tales in the psycho-

logical development of children (cf., Bettelheim, 1977). The intrinsic interest which folktales have for children and the tales' retention of indigenous
cultural values make them a worthy therapeutic tool.

Underlying the development of cuento therapy is the assumption that
the psychological distress experienced by many children who grow up within an alien culture is partly due to a weakened cultural value system, a sense
of distance from the surrounding society, lack of pride in their own ethnic
roots, and the family's diminished role as a cultural agent of socialization.
Folktales are vehicles for the transmission of cultural values and pride. The
ego strengths likely to be weakened through the acculturative process could
thus be reinstated or reinforced.

Some of the children who participated in the study were told Puerto
Rican folktales as they appeared in scholarly listings without alteration. For
these children, an isomorphic relationship was established, the therapy directly mirroring the clients' cultural background. However, since the value
of such an isomorphic relationship was viewed as a hypothesis and not as
an axiom, other children were told folktales which had been changed in
order to convey the knowledge, values and skills deemed useful in coping
with the demands of the sociocultural environment of New York City.

A sample of over 200 Puerto Rican children were identified as a high-risk
group based on their maladaptive behavior in school, their single-parent
households, and low socioeconomic status. The children participated in either an isomorphic or non-isomorphic folktale therapy group, a traditional
therapy group, or a group with no therapeutic intervention. Small groups
of children and their mothers participated in 20 weekly 90-minute therapy
sessions, and all children were pre- and post-tested with a battery of therapeutic outcome measures. In the folktale sessions, two stories were read by
the mothers, and the children followed the narration by listening or reading
silently. Therapists then led a discussion about the meaning of the stories,
analyzing the various behaviors depicted. Then the folktale was dramatized
by the children and their mothers and the skit was videotaped. The dramati-
zation was played back on videotape, and the group therapist emphasized
the maladaptive and adaptive consequences of the behaviors dramatized.

In the traditional group therapy, children and their mothers participated
in a series of recreational tasks under the supervision of the therapist. In
some cases the games were competitive, while in others cooperation between group members was stressed. Psychodrama was also used as group
members enacted common family themes with emphasis placed on their
interpersonal conflicts. As in folktale therapy, the skit was videotaped and
played back for group discussion, eliciting information about participants'

reactions to the family conflict and alternative solutions to lessen family tensions.

Two questions can be posed from this study, one relevant to the first research problem in this chapter and another relevant to the second research problem. First, was the impact of the therapy, whether based on folktales which preserved Puerto Rican culture or on folktales which were modified to bridge Puerto Rican and Anglo culture, different from that of the traditional art/play and non-intervention group? Second, did the adapted folktales have an effect different from that of the original folktales?

The result of the evaluation of therapeutic outcomes was that, in answer to the first question, the two culturally sensitive therapy groups evidenced significantly lower trait anxiety compared to traditional group therapy and non-intervention. Children in the adapted folktale group were rated lower in anxiety than children undergoing original folktale therapy, traditional group therapy, and no therapy. Children in the original folktale group, in turn, were rated as less anxious than children in the non-intervention group, but did not differ from children in the traditional therapy group. Evaluation one year after the termination of therapy showed that this pattern of results was stable, with the exception that the adapted folktale group did not differ significantly from the original folktale group. Given its more immediate impact, the adapted folktale therapy appears to be a more promising technique than a traditional approach or even original folktale therapy. The impact of adapted folktale therapy on trait anxiety is especially compelling since many clinicians concur that prolonged anxiety predisposes individuals to many common forms of psychopathology and also because anxiety disorders are presented frequently by Hispanics at community mental health facilities (Reubens, 1980). The evaluation of folktale therapy with respect to amelioration of symptoms of trait anxiety suggests that altering the therapeutic modality in the direction of the host society is a more effective treatment strategy. Thus, there is some empirical justification for the development of therapies based upon elements taken from the client's culture and for adapting such elements to the host society. But we have no knowledge of how such elements are mediated by the therapeutic process in their influence on treatment outcomes.

The need to examine the specific effects of culture on treatment outcomes, as mediated by the therapeutic process, was discussed in the presentation of the first research problem. This recommendation for future research, as proposed by Sue and Zane (1987), can be extended to the second research problem. Thus, research should be conducted which links the specific departures from the isomorphic assumption to treatment outcomes through a focus on intervening therapeutic processes. The conduct of process-oriented, therapeutic outcome research on the second research problem would be a revealing contribution to our understanding of how planned departures from isomorphic cultural sensitivity lead or do not lead to therapeutic gains.

Summary

The modification of traditional therapeutic modalities and development of new modalities out of cultural traits relevant to the treatment process are ambitious and difficult tasks. This chapter has posed questions, which remain unanswered, about how cultural sensitivity should be introduced into the therapeutic process. Efforts to render therapeutic modalities culturally sensitive, no matter how persuasive or attractive, must ultimately attend to the objectives of maintaining the client in therapy, increasing satisfaction with the therapeutic interchange, and ultimately relieving the client of psychological distress so that an adaptive level of functioning in society is achieved. It should no longer be sufficient for a clinician to merely assert cultural sensitivity based on good intentions alone: as an alternative, we invite our colleagues to situate their clinical innovations into the research problems developed in this chapter. Thus, we invite our colleagues to attend to the distinction we have drawn between isomorphic reinforcement of culture and departures from isomorphism in the interest of the client's well-being.

To attend to such issues, research must be conducted. As Padilla et al. (1975) stated, ". . . an innovative treatment program is self-defeating unless validating research is conducted . . . to guide the development of programs with the greatest probability of success" (p. 900). It is particularly important that innovative modalities not become immersed in the vast pool of other untested therapy modalities. Future research needs to confirm whether cultural sensitivity is a worthwhile aim in providing psychotherapeutic services to Hispanics, and how treatment selections or modifications based on cultural considerations facilitate achieving specific therapeutic goals. On the other hand, the task of evaluation should not deter us from the attempt to explore new culturally sensitive therapeutic alternatives.

References

Acosta, F.X., Evans, L.A., Yamamoto, J. and Wilcox, S.A. (1980). Helping minority and low-income psychotherapy patients "Tell It Like It Is." *Journal of Biocommunication* 7(3): 13-19.

Baekland, F. and Lundwell, L. (1975). Dropping out of treatment: A critical review. *Psychological Bulletin* 82: 738-783.

Bettelheim, B. (1977). *The Uses of Enchantment: The Importance and Meaning of Fairy Tales.* New York: Vintage Books.

Bluestone, H. and Vela, R.M. (1982). Transcultural aspects in the psychotherapy of the Puerto Rican poor in New York City. *Journal of the American Academy of Psychoanalysis* 10: 269-283.

Boulette, T.R. (1976). Assertive training with low-income Mexican American women. In M.R. Miranda (Ed.), *Psychotherapy with the Spanish-Speaking: Issues in Research and Service Delivery.* Los Angeles: University of California, Spanish-Speaking Mental Health Research Center.

Cohen, R.E. (1972). Principles of preventive mental health programs for ethnic minority populations: The acculturation of Puerto Ricans to the United States. *American Journal of Psychiatry* 128: 1529-1533.

Costantino, G., Malgady, R.G. and Rogler, L.H. (1986). Cuento therapy: A culturally sensitive modality for Puerto Rican children. *Journal of Consulting and Clinical Psychology* 54: 639-645.

Eysenck, H. (1952). The effects of psychotherapy: An evaluation. *Journal of Consulting Psychology* 16: 319-324.

Farber, A. and Rogler, L.H. (1981). *Unitas: Hispanic and Black Children in a Healing Community.* New York: Hispanic Research Center, Fordham University (Monograph No. 6).

Garfield, S.L. (1981). Psychotherapy: A forty-year appraisal. *American Psychologist* 36: 174-183.

Gomez, E. (1983). The San Antonio model: A culture-oriented approach. In G. Gibson (Ed.), *Our Kingdom Stands on Brittle Glass.* Silver Springs, Md.: National Association of Social Workers.

Kreisman, J.J. (1975). The curandero's apprentice: A therapeutic integration of folk and medicinal healing. *American Journal of Psychiatry* 132: 81-83.

Luborsky, L., Singler, B. and Luborsky, L. (1975). Comparative studies of psychotherapies. *Archives of General Psychiatry* 32: 995-1008.

Maduro, R.J. and Martinez, C.F. (1974) Latino dream analysis: Opportunity for confrontation. *Social Casework* 55: 461-469.

Maldonado-Sierra, E.D. and Trent, R.D. (1960). The sibling relationship in group psychotherapy with Puerto Rican schizophrenics. *American Journal of Psychiatry* 117: 239-244.

Minuchin, S., Montalvo, B. and Guerney, B. (1967). *Families of the Slums: An Exploration of their Treatment.* New York: Basic Books.

Miranda, M.R. (1976). *Psychotherapy with the Spanish-Speaking: Issues in Research and Service Delivery.* Los Angeles: Spanish-Speaking Mental Health Research Center, University of California (Monograph No. 3).

Padilla, A.M., Ruiz, R.A. and Alvarez, R. (1975). Community mental health services for the Spanish-speaking/surnamed populations. *American Psychologist* 30: 892-905.

Paul, G.L. (1967). Strategy of outcome research in psychotherapy. *Journal of Consulting Psychology* 31: 109-118.

Pitta, P., Marcos, L.R. and Alpert, M. (1978). Language switching as a treatment strategy with bilingual patients. *American Journal of Psychoanalysis* 38: 255-258.

Procidano, M.E. and Glenwick, D.S. (1985). *Unitas: Evaluating a Preventive Program for Hispanic and Black Youth.* New York: Hispanic Research Center, Fordham University (Monograph No. 13).

Reubens, P. (1980). Psychological needs of the new immigrants. *Migration Today* 8(2): 8-14.

Rogler, L.H. and Hollingshead, A.B. (1985). *Trapped: Puerto Rican Families and Schizophrenia,* 3rd ed. Maplewood, N.J.: Waterfront Press.

Rogler, L.H., Malgady, R.G., Costantino, G. and Blumenthal, R. (1987). What do culturally sensitive mental health services mean? The case of Hispanics. *American Psychologist* 42: 565-570.

Ruiz, R. (1981). Cultural and historical perspectives in counseling Hispanics. In D.W. Sue (Ed.), *Counseling the Culturally Different: Theory and Practice.* New York: Wiley and Sons.

Ruiz, R. and Casas, M.E. (1981). Culturally relevant and behaviorist counseling for Chicano college students. In P.P. Pederson et. al. (Eds.), *Counseling across Cultures.* Hawaii: East-West Center.

Smith, M.L. and Glass, G.V. (1977). Meta-analysis of psychotherapy outcome studies. *American Psychologist* 32: 752-760.

Sue, D.W. (Ed.) (1981). *Counseling the Culturally Different: Theory and Practice.* New York: Wiley and Sons.

Sue, S. (1988). Psychotherapeutic services for ethnic minorities. *American Psychologist* 43: 301-308.

Sue S. and Zane, N. (1987). The role of culture and cultural techniques in psychotherapy: A critique and reformulation. *American Psychologist* 42: 37-45.

Szapocznik, J., Scopetta, M.A. and King, O.E. (1978). Theory and practice in matching treatment to the special characteristics and problems of Cuban immigrants. *Journal of Community Psychology* 6: 112-122.

Szapocznik, J., Kurtines, W. and Fernandez, T. (1980). Bicultural involvement and adjustment in Hispanic American youths. *International Journal of Intercultural Relations* 4: 353-365.

Chapter 6

Phase Five: Post-Treatment Adjustment

Mr. Roberto Ruiz recalls that one afternoon twenty years ago when he returned home from his job in a lumber yard, he found his wife looking distraught, hurling pots and pans and music records on the floor, his two children fearfully cowering in their bedroom. He contacted his wife's aunt who lived nearby and was told that previously in Puerto Rico his wife had been hospitalized for a nervous attack. The aunt took care of his children while he took his wife to the psychiatric ward of a local hospital. He dreaded visiting his wife. He recalls a patient in the ward who went through strange motions with her hands. When asked what she was doing, she said she was knitting a sweater for her baby. Later, when the lady was about to be discharged, he asked her if she had finished the baby sweater. The lady replied, "What sweater? I have no baby." It bothered him to have his wife in a place with crazy persons, and, along with his children, he was relieved when she returned home.

A year later, his wife's brother died in Puerto Rico and he, himself, lost his job in the lumber yard. Then at three o'clock one morning his wife began to alternate uncontrollably between laughing and weeping. He felt he could not cope with his wife's illness again. He woke up his children who were reluctant to get up, dressed them, and made his wife get dressed. With a child under each arm, he nudged and pushed his wife forward to the subway station. But the train rushed by without his being able to carry out his plan of hurling everyone, including himself, on the tracks. He returned home, asked a neighbor to take care of the children and took his wife again to the psychiatric ward of the hospital.

* * *

The fifth and last phase of the framework's temporal sequence begins after the client terminates therapy. In this phase the person faces a new set of potentially problematic questions such as how well he or she will be able to resume customary social roles within the family and the work place, and whether the continued support of mental health professionals, family mem-

119

bers, and others will be needed to sustain the person as a functioning member of the community. Depending on the seriousness and prognosis of the illness, treatment may have involved one or two visits to an outpatient setting or an extended period of hospitalization. Whether outpatient or inpatient, all therapies examine interpersonal relationships between the client and the family. Therefore, upon termination of the treatment, family members may face adjustments of their relationships in line with the therapist's advice. Post-treatment adjustment is particularly problematic to the chronically or seriously mentally ill (SMI), i.e., persons whose illness produces life disruptions so great as to require periods of hospitalization. Although applicable to a variety of psychiatric diagnoses and to substance-use problems, this type of distress is often associated with psychoses, such as schizophrenia, and severe affective disorders.

There are two research problems in Phase Five, both concerning Hispanic SMI's post-treatment adjustment problems. The first focuses upon the Hispanic patient's reintegration into the family and community; the second examines Hispanics' use of post-treatment services. However, before we discuss these problems, it would be informative to review briefly the sociodemographic and mental health policy changes which have highlighted the importance of the research problems selected.

During the last two decades, the SMI's post-treatment problems have been nationally recognized as mental health facilities began to deinstitutionalize their long-term patient populations. Mental health policy in the 1960's assumed that deinstitutionalization would be accompanied by improvements in the efficacy of psychotropic medication and the expansion of social and mental health programs. Proposals were made to increase the number of community residences such as half-way houses as alternatives to institutionalization, and to develop community mental health centers to treat the SMI on an outpatient basis. Indeed, annual admissions to state hospitals decreased from 390,000 in 1972, when 64 percent of the cases were readmissions (Special Populations Sub-Task Panel on Mental Health of Hispanic Americans, 1978) to 369,049 in 1980, when 80 percent were readmissions (Rosenstein et al., 1987). The fact that in the last two decades high rates of deinstitutionalization have been combined with high rates of readmissions suggests that deinstitutionalization was not accompanied by highly effective social and mental health programs. As Bessuk and Gerson (1978) assert, despite the promise of treatment and rehabilitation embodied in the community mental health programs, deinstitutionalization has often meant hardship and tragedy to the thousands of hospitalized patients released haphazardly to a "non-system of community aftercare." Many of these individuals, discharged after long periods of custodial care, lead a marginal existence in the community, surviving on welfare payments, perhaps receiving some medication or counseling. Unable to cope, they return to the hospital to be maintained on antipsychotic medication. Goldstein's (1981) observation that 85 percent of the patients discharged as a result of deinstitutionalization are located in the lower or working classes adds poignancy to the problem.

Mechanic (1988) points out that the deleterious effects of deinstitutionalization have been exacerbated by the changing demography of the American population, namely, the growth of the older-age population and the fact that the great numbers of the "baby-boom" population reached adulthood in the 1970's. The latter fact has increased the number of people in the age group when schizophrenia is most likely to develop. This is particularly relevant for Hispanic mental health because the Hispanic population is one of the youngest in the United States. Nationally, the median age for Hispanics is 23.2, in contrast to a median age of 30.4 for non-Hispanics (U.S. Census, 1980). Their age characteristics suggest that Hispanics will constitute a significant portion of the schizophrenic population in the near future, and that post-treatment adjustment is an important Hispanic mental health issue.

In addition to changes in the age structure, changes in the family structure may well pose post-treatment problems for Hispanics. The research literature points to the importance Hispanics ascribe to the solidarity of family relationships (Rogler, 1978; Rogler and Cooney, 1984). However, consistent with trends for the population as a whole, the Hispanic family has become increasingly subject to strains, as indicated by its high female-head-of-household rate. For example, in 1960, 15.8 percent of Puerto Rican families were female-headed, while in 1980, 34.8 percent were female-headed (Tienda and Jensen, 1986). Taken in conjunction with other trends, such as the increase in teenage pregnancy among Hispanics, a picture emerges of individuals not being able to rely as fully as they did previously on the instrumental and emotional supports traditionally provided by the family. Furthermore, since the expanded system of community health care which accompanied deinstitutionalization did not absorb the newly discharged clients, mental health policy implicitly assumed the family to be the primary medium for custodial care of the SMI.

If this assumption about the family is juxtaposed with the increased strains and dissolutions experienced by families in the last three decades, clearly post-treatment adjustment is highly problematic for Hispanics and other low socioeconomic groups. Nonetheless, there is little information to shed light on these problems. When the framework presented in this book was first published (Rogler et al., 1983), the post-treatment experiences of Hispanics were singled out as the most neglected area of Hispanic mental health research. Five years later, Padilla et al.'s (1988) examination of the issue made the same observation. This paucity of information should be kept in mind during our examination of the pertinent literature below.

The two research problems which we will discuss in this phase correspond to two major dimensions of the Hispanic post-treatment experience—reintegration into the family and community and the use of post-treatment services. Both dimensions aim to prevent the recurrence of serious psychological distress and consequent rehospitalization, but they operate in different settings: the first primarily in the family and community, and the second in the mental health system. Therefore, each dimension is treated as a separate research problem, although some explanatory factors are possibly common to both.

The first research problem concerns the applicability to Hispanics of proposals made in the general rehabilitation literature. In considering post-treatment reintegration into the family and community, this literature asserts that lower socioeconomic status and life-event stresses are linked to difficulties in post-treatment adjustment; attributes of social networks, such as size, are associated with positive post-treatment experiences; and the family's adjustment to the SMI has a bearing upon the patient's relapse and rehospitalization rates. How applicable are these assertions to the post-treatment experience of Hispanics? The importance of the first problem is based on the conclusion that current research provides no clear answer to this question.

The second research problem delves into Hispanics' use of post-treatment services. The issue lends itself to the formulations concerning alternative resource and barrier theories, discussed in Chapter 3, which sought to explain variations in Hispanics' use of mental health services. However, additional issues have to be considered in this phase of the framework, such as the scarcity of aftercare mental health services and the lack of continuity between treatment and aftercare services.

Family and Community Reintegration

In assessing the post-treatment level of functioning of the SMI, the two most often used criteria are rehospitalization and employment. The assumption behind the first measure is that rehospitalization signals the individual's difficulties in adjusting to the role requirements of living in a family and in the community. Behind the second criterion is the assumption that the employed individual is less likely to be a financial burden to the family and to society, and is evidencing a capacity for some level of functioning. The sociodemographic and mental health policy changes discussed earlier in this chapter suggest that resumption of family roles is an additional criterion of post-treatment adjustment. The first research problem considers the relevance to SMI Hispanics of factors that the research literature has associated with post-treatment adjustment. Before examining these factors, it is necessary to consider the relevance of rehospitalization, employment, and family reintegration to the situation of Hispanics.

Since the absence of rehospitalization is considered a major indicator of successful post-treatment adjustment, a useful starting point would be to compare Hispanics' rehospitalization rates with those of other groups. As indicated earlier, approximately two-thirds of admissions to state hospitals are readmissions of previously hospitalized persons (Special Populations Sub-Task Panel, 1978). Goering et al. (1984) estimated that one-third of discharged patients are readmitted to inpatient facilities within two months and two-thirds within two years. Unfortunately, comparative information on the rehospitalization rates of different ethnic groups is not available. Such information is crucial in order to assess the seriousness of Hispanics' post-treatment adjustment problems. The discussion of mental health utilization rates in Chapter 3 also points to the need to collect information on the proportion of SMI persons requiring but not receiving hospitalization.

Employment, used as an indicator of post-treatment adjustment, is a critical variable on several levels: it is an indication that a person can function at least minimally; it is an aid to rehabilitation; and it provides evidence of wellness (Wansbrough and Cooper, 1980). Serban and Thomas (1974) have linked rehospitalization to unemployment and dependence on public assistance. The significance of work in interpreting the post-treatment adjustment of clients very likely depends upon the socioeconomic level and the cultural group's normative orientation toward work and other institutional structures. Among Hispanics such issues remain unexamined, but it is possible that for many SMI Hispanics the inability to find gainful employment may be as much a function of low socioeconomic status, disadvantaged status in the labor market, and downturns in the economic cycle as it is a function of psychological impairment.

The resumption of family roles also requires consideration. At minimum, it is important to know what proportion of patients living with their families before hospitalization return to those families after discharge, and how Hispanics compare to other groups in this proportion. The presence of disturbed homeless persons in the streets of major cities suggests that a substantial proportion of the SMI do not return to their families after discharge and are homeless. Pepper and Ryglewicz (1982) found that 23 percent of patients released in New York State in 1975 went to live with relatives, 38 percent went to boarding houses, single-room-occupancy dwellings or hotels, and 11 percent went to nursing homes. The remaining 28 percent vanished from the records, suggesting that they became homeless or transients in different kinds of living arrangements. Sadly, resumption of family roles appears to be the exception for SMI clients released from psychiatric facilities, and there is no reason to expect that Hispanics have a different pattern.

For those who return to their families after terminating treatment, little is known about the nature of reintegration into the family. A fairly large literature focusing upon post-treatment therapeutic modalities suggests important dimensions of family reintegration, such as regaining the skills necessary for daily functioning (Goldstein, 1981). Obviously, performing elementary activities such as shopping and using public transportation is an important aspect of reintegration into the family. However, it will be seen below that other, more subtle, social psychological aspects of family reintegration need to be considered, for example, the extent to which the discharged patient displays behavior which increases intrafamilial stress.

Now that the multidimensional nature of family and community reintegration has been highlighted, the discussion will turn to those factors that the research literature associates with post-treatment adjustment. Socioeconomic status has long been recognized as a major factor. More recently, life-event stress, family relationships, and social network influences have also been posited to influence post-treatment adjustment. The first research problem considers how these factors may influence the post-treatment adjustment of SMI Hispanics.

Socioeconomic status, as we have seen in the previous phases of the conceptual framework, plays a fundamental role in the client's experience of the mental health system. Social class continues to be a major factor in what happens after treatment as well. Thus, Zigler and Phillips (1960), using case history data to predict aftercare outcome for discharged schizophrenics, found that a high occupational and educational status, a good employment history, and being married before hospitalization are variables which predict a favorable outcome upon discharge. In Myers and Bean's (1968) follow-up study of Hollingshead and Redlich's investigation of social class and mental illness, the deleterious results of being both seriously disturbed and a member of the lower class are strikingly documented. Lower class clients are more likely than the affluent to be readmitted to the hospital, and those who are not rehospitalized are more likely than higher class clients to experience employment difficulties, financial problems, and extreme social isolation. Myers and Bean's thesis is that the lower the social class, the more severely handicapping is the role of the mental patient. The relationship between social class and post-treatment adjustment within the Hispanic community remains unknown.

A number of researchers have studied the role of environmental stress on post-treatment adjustment. Brown and Birley (1968) indicate that the risk of schizophrenic relapse increases during the three weeks following a stressful life event. Keeping in mind the previous discussion of the relation between social class and rehospitalization risk, as well as the discussion in Chapter 2 about the role of life-event stress in creating psychological distress among Hispanics, one would expect that the Hispanic SMI client, being at the lower end of the socioeconomic scale, is more likely than members of more affluent groups to experience stress and therefore be more vulnerable to relapse.

Isolation of the SMI and their family members from supportive networks of relatives and friends has also been considered an important factor in post-treatment adjustment (Anderson et al., 1980; Atwood and Williams, 1978; Beels, 1975). Isolation is likely to occur in segments of the population who experience migration and the stresses of acculturation (Hammer, 1981). Such isolation promotes withdrawal, which frequently foreshadows the onset of a schizophrenic episode. Gittleman-Klein and Klein (1969) found a strong association between poor outcome and restricted premorbid social contacts. Strauss and Carpenter (1972, 1974) show that the amount of social contact just prior to hospitalization served as a strong predictor of outcome five years later, while an earlier study by Hammer (1963-64) also found that network variables were associated with the likelihood of rehospitalization among schizophrenic patients. Several recent studies have compared the immediate networks of schizophrenics with those of non-psychotic individuals and have reported smaller networks for schizophrenics than for those in remission or for those who never had the illness (Pattison et al., 1979; Sokolovsky et al., 1978). Garrison (1978) found an inverse relationship between network size and rehospitalization rates among Puerto Rican women in New York City. Network characteristics other than size have also been associated with post-treatment outcomes. Hammer (1961, 1963-1964) found that schizophrenics in closed networks—those where friends and family members know each other—have lower rehospitalization rates than those in open networks. Pattison (1979) and Tolsdorf (1976) found that schizophrenics' networks are more likely than those of non-schizophrenics to be restricted to family members.

The isolation of schizophrenics and their families assumes greater significance when one considers the important functions of social networks. Among these functions, Hammer (1981) emphasizes social and instrumental support, access to others, information exchange and mediation between the family and the sick person, all of which are necessary for coping with an SMI client. On the other hand, Leff (1976) and Garrison (1978) believe that contact with families is often deleterious for discharged clients. However, as Dean and Lin's (1977) review of the literature concludes, lack of social support significantly increases vulnerability to ordinary stressors in both medical and psychiatric illness.

Much of the current post-treatment adjustment research focuses upon interpersonal relations in families with SMI individuals. Creer and Wing (1974) and Hatfield (1978) describe the behaviors of discharged schizophrenics that their families view as disturbing and problematical. Among these are social withdrawal, uncommunicativeness, inappropriate affect, lack of leisure interests, and delusional ideas. These social deficits impose burdens on family members because they indicate that their relative is unable to meet family expectations such as providing companionship and displaying affection. In turn, the family's reaction to the SMI member's inability to meet their expectations may adversely influence the latter's prognosis. Families may precipitate specific episodes of disturbed behavior, thereby contributing to the client's relapse and rehospitalization (Bateson et al., 1956; Lidz, 1973; Wynne and Singer, 1963; Singer and Wynne, 1965). Zwerling and Mendelsohn (1965) show that when families regard the patients' difficulties as symptoms rather than as evidence of weak character, the prognosis for avoidance of rehospitalization improves. Other studies show that the higher the family's expectations about the patient's ability to carry out customary family roles, the greater the avoidance of rehospitalization (Carpenter and Boureston, 1976; Freeman and Simmons, 1963; Michaux et al., 1969). Therefore, the family's reaction to the returning patient has several dimensions, and high expectations about the returning patients are not necessarily incompatible with viewing the patient's difficulties as symptoms of the illness.

Another approach to post-treatment adjustment focuses upon the concept of expressed emotion (EE) by family members as a predictor of relapse into schizophrenia. EE is defined as the expression of attitudes towards the client's mental illness, such as criticism of the client's illness-related behavior by family members (Brown et al., 1962; Leff, 1976; Leff and Vaughn, 1981; Vaughn and Leff, 1976). Studies show that clients with high EE families relapse significantly more than those with low EE families. Karno (in

Goldstein and Doane, 1982) found a lower incidence of EE among Mexican Americans than among non-Mexican Americans. This may mean that some Hispanic groups have low EE and indirectly lower the risk of rehospitalization among SMI Hispanics. However, more information is needed about the concept of EE in relation to the diversity of Hispanic groups.

These findings support the rationale for the psychoeducational approach to post-therapy treatment of the SMI (Anderson et al., 1980; Goldstein and Kopeikin, 1983; Faloon et al., 1982, 1987; Leff et al., 1982; McFarlane, 1982) which attempts to provide family members with information about the origin of schizophrenia and other serious mental illnesses, and give them concrete advice about how to adapt their behavior and attitudes toward the client so as to diminish family stresses. However, there is little research on Hispanic families with respect to these issues. Rogler and Hollingshead (1985) and Amin (1974) provide some clues about factors that may influence the adjustment of SMI Hispanic families. The former study pointed out that lower class Puerto Rican families are better able to adjust to a schizophrenic father than a schizophrenic mother, because wives are more central to the emotional structure of such families than husbands. Amin suggests that traditional Hispanic values, such as familism, aids the adjustment of the family to the client's illness and could offset the disruptive effects of low socioeconomic status and stress. In research designed to evaluate the impact of an aftercare program for SMI Hispanics, Rodriguez (1985) found that the families view good relations between the client and the family as more problematic than the clients' inadequate daily living skills. Based on her observations of psychoeducational groups conducted among minority families of discharged schizophrenics, and in keeping with the discussion of cultural sensitivity in Chapter 5, Rivera (1988) suggested that certain elements of treatment, such as the emphasis on egalitarian decision-making, may require modification to make them more applicable to traditionally oriented Hispanic families. Limited as these findings are, they suggest that attention must be paid to the cultural aspects of Hispanic social life, such as role prescriptions for males and females, and family norms and values, and generally to acculturation. With respect to these and other issues, there is a great need for studies that identify how the process of family and community reintegration occurs among Hispanics. However, for the SMI, successful adjustment involves not only return to the family and community, but also the use of aftercare services, vocational rehabilitation and other types of services. The next research problem turns to the Hispanic experience in using these services.

The Use of Post-Treatment Services

In addition to examining the impact of variables such as stress, social networks, and family relationships on post-treatment adjustment, some researchers have examined the adequacy of services provided to psychiatric clients after discharge from treatment, and the role of the mental health system in inducing compliance with aftercare plans. These issues assume critical importance in helping clients and their families to cope with problems of reintegration into the community. The second research problem concerns those factors influencing SMI Hispanics' use of these services. Before discussing this, the types and availability of post-treatment services will be briefly reviewed.

A discharge plan is routinely constructed when a client is about to be discharged from treatment. The plan considers whether or not the client is likely to return to the family, the desirability of other living arrangements, and the type of aftercare services needed by the client. Upon termination of treatment, most SMI face the options of either returning to the family, living alone—often in inadequate housing, or homelessness. For a small minority, discharge is followed by community residential treatment such as group living in a half-way house or foster-care placements with families not related to the client. Although the development of community living arrangements was emphasized by the deinstitutionalization movement and the expansion of social programs in the 1960's and 1970's, they comprise only a small part of aftercare for the SMI. Rare as these services are, however, they are an alternative for clients without families or with troublesome family situations. Little is known about the number of SMI Hispanics who are placed in community living arrangements or about the post-treatment experiences of those who are.

Vocational rehabilitation is another kind of aftercare service for the SMI. Given their relatively poor labor market prospects and low socioeconomic status, SMI Hispanics, it would appear, could derive benefits from vocational rehabilitation. However, vocational rehabilitation has traditionally excluded the SMI (Torrey, 1983). The U.S. Department of Labor's main focus has been the poorly educated, while the U.S. Department of Health and Human Services concentrates its programs on the physically handicapped. Considering the need, there are few programs to rehabilitate the SMI who are capable of returning to work, and little is known about the number of Hispanics placed in this type of service and its impact on their post-treatment adjustment.

In contrast to community living arrangements and vocational rehabilitation, outpatient treatment is the primary aftercare service for the SMI. An important objective of outpatient treatment is to monitor the client's compliance with the medication regimen, since treatment with psychotropic medicines requires frequent monitoring over long periods of time by someone who is familiar with the client. The utility of aftercare is supported by Anthony's research (1980) which found that clients treated in aftercare clinics had lower hospitalization rates than those receiving other types of treatment such as follow-up counseling. However, other studies question the effectiveness of these services for most clients. Two studies tracked cohorts of clients discharged from psychiatric hospitals through an entire mental health aftercare system and found that most clients made contact with some type of aftercare service within one year after discharge, but that the typical patterns were of short-term contacts with multiple agencies rather than sustained contact with one agency (Goering et al., 1984; Solomon et al., 1983). In addition, the research found more reliance on medical services than on other components of aftercare. For example, when the needs for housing, recreation, vocational, and educational services were identified, referrals for such services were infrequently made by discharge planners. Thus, although most clients are in contact with the aftercare system, the primary services offered are maintenance-oriented rather than rehabilitation-oriented. At best, such services may stabilize the clients temporarily and provide them with some social support, but the services are not likely to provide social and vocational training or to reduce long-term dependence of the patients or maximize their functioning.

The above-mentioned studies were conducted in Toronto and in the states of Washington and Idaho. The aftercare system in the inner-city neighborhoods where Hispanics reside may be even less responsive. In an evaluation of a South Bronx demonstration project for SMI Hispanics, Rodriguez (1985) found that two-fifths of the persons in a designated catchment area who had been released from the local state hospital did not seek aftercare, nor did 70 percent of Hispanic patients released from the area's general hospital's short-term psychiatric ward and referred to aftercare. While it is possible that some of these clients sought services in other catchment areas, it is more probable that the majority did not receive any type of mental health care after discharge. The study raises doubts about the extent to which Hispanic and other low-income minority SMI clients make use of or are linked with aftercare services.

What factors account for SMI Hispanics' utilization of aftercare services? It could be that aftercare utilization is a special case of the general problem of how psychologically distressed Hispanics seek help, which was discussed in Chapter 3. There we found two major explanations of underutilization: alternative resource theory and barrier theory. Briefly recounting the theories: alternative resource theory states that Hispanics underutilize mental health services because they rely for counseling on informal group structures such as the family, friendship networks, and spiritualists; in contrast, barrier theory posits two types of obstacles to the use of mental health services—cultural values and norms which make Hispanics reluctant to use bureaucratically run professional mental health services and institutional barriers such as the lack of Spanish-speaking professionals in agencies, which make these services inaccessible to Hispanics. The second research problem examines the applicability of these explanations to aftercare mental health services.

Do families, neighbors and spiritualists provide alternatives to use of aftercare clinics and other post-treatment services? A positive answer is plausible. For example, Rogler and Hollingshead (1985) showed that sometimes Puerto Rican families took their schizophrenic family members to spiritualists to address the causes of the illnesses and to psychiatrists to relieve the symptoms. In some cases, the psychiatrists were used to calm the afflicted family member so that he or she could be taken to a spiritualist. Similarly, explanations of underutilization based on cultural and institutional barriers also are plausible and, equally, there is little information to verify them. The research literature examined in Chapter 3 indicates a positive relationship between acculturation level and services utilization (c.f. Edgerton and Karno, 1971; Rodriguez, 1987). Rodriguez's finding (1986) that unacculturated Hispanic clients of an aftercare clinic were more likely than the acculturated to drop out of treatment is also relevant to the utilization of aftercare services.

Rivera (1986) discusses a number of institutional barriers specific to use of aftercare services by SMI Hispanics. Among these are the fragmentation of services, particularly the tenuous links between inpatient and aftercare facilities, which often leads to discharged clients not being placed in aftercare (Barrow et al., 1979; Goering et al., 1984; Hargreaves, 1988; Solomon et al., 1983); the lack of interest by community mental health centers in treating the SMI and the failure to provide consistent aftercare (Beiser et al., 1985; Solomon et al., 1983; Torrey, 1983); and the lack of social support services such as half-way houses (Pepper and Ryglewicz, 1982; Torrey, 1983) and vocational rehabilitation (Serban and Thomas, 1974; Talbot, 1978; Torrey, 1983). It is important to note that these studies address the needs of the SMI population in general, not specifically those of Hispanics. Critical as they are, they do not throw light on institutional barriers of relevance to Hispanic utilization of aftercare programs. However, it should be mentioned that Rodriguez's study (1986), which linked an increase in SMI Hispanic utilization of an aftercare clinic to the overcoming of language and other barriers, is consistent with studies which have found that utilization increases when mental health facilities reduce barriers that keep Hispanics away (c.f., Karno and Morales, 1971; Treviño et al., 1979).

Summary

Two research problems in Phase Five of the hypothetical temporal sequence were examined, along with the relevance to Hispanics of recent changes affecting aftercare reintegration into the family and community. The first problem calls for the identification of factors influencing the discharged client's reintegration into the family and community. The sociodemographic and mental health policy changes previously discussed make post-treatment adjustment a pervasive and complex problem that can no longer be conceived only in terms of resumption of employment and prevention of rehospitalization. Other things must be taken into account, and the gap of our ignorance with respect to Hispanics thus widens. Little is known about rehospitalization rates among Hispanics, the proportion of SMI Hispanics who are employed, and how many return to their families, enter alternative living arrangements, or become homeless after treatment. Lower social class individuals have been shown to have poorer prospects of post-treatment adjustment than more affluent persons, and Hispanics are more than amply represented among the lower and working classes of American society. Life-event stress has been linked to vulnerability to psychological distress and to difficulties in post-treatment adjustment. The life conditions of Hispanics subject them to these stresses more than many other groups. Social network attributes such as size, frequency of interaction, and extent of support provided have been associated with positive post-treatment experiences. However, the few studies of Hispanics pertinent to this issue provide no information on the role of Hispanics' social network in post-treatment adjustment. Finally, family members' adjustment to the behavior of discharged SMI clients and their ability to view the SMI's behavior objectively improve the SMI's chances of avoiding relapse and rehospitalization.

Upon termination of treatment, the SMI may require alternatives to family living, such as group living in a half-way house or foster care placement, and vocational rehabilitation. All discharged patients require aftercare treatment to monitor the psychotropic medications needed to alleviate the illness and to receive counseling when needed. The studies reviewed indicate that vocational rehabilitation and community residential services are scarce, and the few studies available question the effectiveness of aftercare services for most clients. The second research problem considered the applicability of alternative resource and barrier theories to the aftercare utilization of mental health facilities. The theories, plausibly, could be applied. The common denominator in this discussion has been the dearth of research relevant to the Hispanic experience in the post-treatment phase.

References

Amin, A.E. (1974). Culture and Post-Hospital Community Adjustment of Long-Term Hospitalized Puerto Rican Schizophrenic Patients in New York City. (Doctoral dissertation, Columbia University; also *Dissertation Abstracts International* 35, 5964B, University Microfilms #74-26579).

Anderson, C.M., Hogardy, G. and Reiss, D.J. (1980). Family treatment of adult schizophrenic patients: A psychoeducational approach. *Schizophrenia Bulletin* 6: 490-505.

Anthony, W.A. (1980). *The Principles of Psychiatric Rehabilitation.* Baltimore, Md.: University Park Press.

Atwood, N. and Williams, M. (1978). Group support for the families of the mentally ill. *Schizophrenia Bulletin* 4(3): 415-425.

Barrow, S., Gutwirth, L. and Schwartz, C.C. (1979). Aftercare compliance of chronic patients. Paper presented at Annual Meeting of American Psychiatric Association, Chicago.

Bateson, G., Jackson, D.D., Haley, J. and Weakland, J. (1956). Toward a theory of schizophrenia. *Behavioral Science* 1: 251-264.

Beels, C.C. (1975). Family and social management of schizophrenia. *Schizophrenia Bulletin* 1(13): 97-118.

Beiser, M., Shore, J.H., Peters, R. and Tatum, E. (1985). Does community care for the mentally ill make a difference? A tale of two cities. *American Journal of Psychiatry* 142(9): 1047-1052.

Bessuk, E.L. and Gerson, S. (1978). Deinstitutionalization and mental health services. *Scientific American* 238: 46-53.

Brown, G. and Birley, J. (1968) Crises and life changes and the onset of schizophrenia. *Journal of Health and Social Behavior* 9:203-214.

Brown, G.W., Monck, E., Carstairs, G.M. and Wing, J. (1962). Influence of family life in the course of schizophrenic illness. *British Journal of Preventative and Social Medicine* 16:55-68.

Carpenter, J.D. and Boureston, N.C. (1976). Performance of psychiatric hospital discharges in strict and tolerant environments. *Community Mental Health Journal* 12:45-51.

Creer, C., and Wing, J. (1974). *Schizophrenia at Home?* Monograph, London: Institute of Psychiatry.

Dean A., and Lin, N. (1977). The stress-buffering role of social support. *Journal of Nervous and Mental Disease* 165:403-416.

Edgerton R.B. and Karno, M. (1971). Mexican American bilingualism and the perception of mental illness. *Archives of General Psychiatry* 24:286-290.

Faloon, I., Boyd, J.L., McGill, C., Razoni, J., Moss, H.B. and Gilderman H.M. (1982). Family management in the prevention of exacerbations of schizophrenia: A controlled study. *New England Journal of Medicine* 306: 1437-1440.

Faloon, I., Boyd, J.L., McGill, C., Strang, J., and Moss, H. (1987). Family management training in the community care of schizophrenia. In M.J. Goldstein (Ed.) *New Developments in Interventions with Families of Schizophrenics.* San Francisco: Jossey-Bass.

Freeman, H. and Simmons, O. (1963). *The Mental Patient Comes Home.* New York: Wiley and Sons.

Garrison, V. (1978). Puerto Rican women in New York City. *Schizophrenia Bulletin* 4: 561-596.

Gittleman-Klein, R., and Klein, D.F. (1969). Premorbid asocial adjustment and prognosis in schizophrenia. *Journal of Psychiatric Research* 7: 35-53.

Goering, P., Wasylenski, D., Lancee, W., and Freeman, S. (1984). From hospital to community: Six-month and two-year outcomes for 505 patients. *Journal of Nervous and Mental Diseases* 172: 667-673.

Goldstein, A.P. (1981). *Psychological Training: The Structured Technique.* New York: Pergamon Press.

Goldstein, M.J. and Doane, J.A. (1982). Family factors in the onset, course, and treatment of schizophrenic spectrum disorders: An update on current research. *Journal of Nervous and Mental Disease* 170: 692-700.

Goldstein, M.J. and Kopeikin, H. (1981). Stress and long-term effects of combining drug and family therapy. In M.J. Goldstein (Ed.). *New Developments in Interventions with Families of Schizophrenics.* San Francisco: Jossey-Bass.

Hammer M. (1961). An Analysis of Social Networks as Factors Influencing the Hospitalization of Mental Patients. Ph.D. dissertation, Columbia University. *Dissertation Abstracts International.* Ann Arbor, Michigan: University Microfilms 61(3383).

Hammer M. (1963-1964). Influence of small social networks as factors in mental hospital admission. *Human Organization* 22: 243-251.

Hammer M. (1981). Social support, social networks, and schizophrenia. *Schizophrenia Bulletin* 7: 45-57.

Hargreaves, W.A. (1988). Three Treatment Systems: Case Management of the Severely Disabled. Paper presented at the Conference on Mental Health Services for the Seriously Mentally Ill: Fostering Useful Knowledge, University of California, Los Angeles.

Hatfield, A.B. (1975). Psychological costs of schizophrenia to the family. *Social Work* (Sept): 355-359.

Karno, M. and Morales, A. (1971). A community mental health service for Mexican Americans in a metropolis. *Comprehensive Psychiatry* 12: 116-121.

Leff, J.P. (1976). Schizophrenia and sensitivity to the family environment. *Schizophrenia Bulletin* 2: 566-574.

Leff, J.P. and Vaughn, C. (1981). The role of maintenance therapy and relatives' expressed emotion in relapse of schizophrenia: A two-year follow up. *British Journal of Psychiatry* 139: 102-104.

Leff, J.P., Kurpers, L., Berkowitz, R., Eberlain-Vries, R. and Sturgeon, D. (1982). A controlled trial of social intervention in the families of schizophrenic patients. *British Journal of Psychiatry* 141: 121-134.

Lidz, T. (1973). *The Origin and Treatment of Schizophrenic Disorders.* New York: Basic Books.

McFarlane, W.R. (1983). *Family Therapy in Schizophrenia.* New York: Guildford Press.

Mechanic, D. (1988). Recent Developments in Mental Health Perspectives and Services. Paper presented at the Conference on Mental Health Services for the Seriously Mentally Ill: Fostering Useful Knowledge, University of California, Los Angeles.

Michaux, W., Katz, M., Kurland, A. and Gansereit, K. (1969): *The First Year Out: Mental Patients after Hospitalization.* Baltimore: Johns Hopkins Press.

Myers, J.K. and Bean, L.L. (1968). *A Decade Later: A Follow-Up of Social Class and Mental Illness.* New York: Wiley and Sons.

Padilla, A.M., Cervantes, R.C., and Salgado de Snyder, N. (1988). Mental Health Services for the Hispanic Chronic Mentally Ill. Paper presented at the Conference on Mental Health Services for the Seriously Mentally Ill: Fostering Useful Knowledge, University of California, Los Angeles.

Pattison, E.M., Llamas, R. and Hurd, G. (1979). Social network mediation of anxiety. *Psychiatric Annals* 9: 56-67.

Pepper, B. and Ryglewicz, H. (1982). Testimony for the neglected: The mentally ill in the post-deinstitutionalized age. *American Journal of Orthopsychiatry* 52(3): 388-392.

Rivera, C. (1986). Research issues: Post-hospitalization adjustment of chronically mentally ill Hispanic patients. Hispanic Research Center *Research Bulletin,* Vol. 9, No. 1, Fordham University, Bronx, New York.

Rivera, C. (1988). Culturally sensitive aftercare services for chronically mentally ill Hispanics: The case of the psychoeducational approach. Hispanic Research Center *Research Bulletin,* Vol.11, No.1., Fordham University, Bronx, New York.

Rodriguez, O. (1985). Project COPA Evaluation: Final Report. Document, Hispanic Research Center, Fordham University, Bronx, New York.

Rodriguez, O. (1986). Overcoming barriers to clinical services among chronically mentally ill Hispanics: Lessons from the evaluation of the Project COPA demonstration. Hispanic Research Center *Research Bulletin,* Vol. 9, No. 1, Fordham University, Bronx, New York.

Rodriguez, O. (1987). *Hispanics and Human Services: Help-Seeking in the Inner City.* Bronx, New York: Hispanic Research Center, Fordham University (Monograph No. 14).

Rogler, L.H. (1978). Help patterns, the family, and mental health: Puerto Ricans in the United States. *International Migration Review* 14: 193-214.

Rogler, L.H., and Cooney, R.S. (1984). *Puerto Rican Families in New York City: Intergenerational Processes.* Maplewood, NJ: Waterfront Press (Hispanic Research Research Center Monograph No. 11).

Rogler, L.H. and Hollingshead, A.B. (1985). *Trapped: Puerto Rican Families and Schizophrenia,* 3rd ed. Maplewood, N.J.: Waterfront Press.

Rogler, L.H., Santana, R.C., Costantino, G., Earley, B.F., Grossman, B., Gurak, D.T., Malgady, R. and Rodriguez, O. (1983). *A Conceptual Framework for Mental Health Research on Hispanic Populations.* Bronx, New York: Hispanic Research Center, Fordham University (Monograph No. 10).

Rosenstein, M.J., Milazzo-Sayre, L.J., MacAskill, R.L. and Manderscheid, R.W. (1987). Use of inpatient psychiatric services by special populations (pp. 59-97). In R.W. Manderscheid and S.A. Barrett (Eds.). *Mental Health, United States, 1987.* Maryland: National Institute of Mental Health, Division of Biometry and Applied Sciences.

Serban, G. and Thomas, A. (1974). Attitudes and behavior of acute and chronic schizophrenic patients regarding ambulatory treatment. *American Journal of Psychiatry* 131: 991-995.

Singer, M.T. and Wynne, L.C. (1965). Thought disorder and family relations of schizophrenia (III). *Archives of General Psychiatry* 12: 187-212.

Sokolovsky, J., Cohen, C., Berger, D. and George J. (1978). Personal networks of ex-mental patients in a Manhattan SRO hotel. *Human Organization* 37: 5-15.

Soloman, P., Gordon, B. and Davis, J.M. (1983). An assessment of aftercare within a community mental health system. *Psychosocial Rehabilitation Journal* VII(2): 33-39.

Special Populations Sub-Task Panel on Mental Health of Hispanic Americans. (1978). *Report to the President's Commission on Mental Health.* Los Angeles: Spanish-Speaking Mental Health Research Center, University of California, p. 4.

Strauss, J.S. and Carpenter, W.T., Jr. (1972). The prediction of outcome in schizophrenia (I). *Archives of General Psychiatry* 27: 739-746.

Strauss, J.S. and Carpenter, W.T., Jr. (1974). The prediction of outcome in schizophrenia (II). *Archives of General Psychiatry* 31:37-42.

Talbot, J.A. (1978). What are the problems of chronic mental patients: A report of a survey of psychiatrists' concerns (pp. 1-7). In J.A. Talbott (Ed.) *The Chronic Mental Patient.* Washington, D.C.: American Psychiatric Association.

Tienda, M. and Jensen, L. (1986). Poverty and minorities: A quarter-century profile of color and socioeconomic disadvantages. Unpublished Manuscript.

Tolsdorf, C.C. (1976). Social networks, support and coping: An exploratory study. *Family Process* 15(4): 407-417.

Torrey, E.F. (1983). *Surviving Schizophrenia: A Family Manual.* New York: Harper and Row.

Treviño, T.M., Bruhn, J.G. and Bunce, H. III. (1979). Utilization of community mental health services in a Texas-Mexico border city. *Social Sciences and Medicine* 13(3A): 331-334.

U.S. Bureau of the Census. (1980). *Census of Population.* Washington, D.C.: U.S. Government Printing Office.

Vaughn, C. and Leff, L. (1976). The influence of family and social factors on the course of psychiatric illness. *British Journal of Psychiatry* 129: 125-137.

Wansbrough, N. and Cooper, P. (1980). *Open Employment After Mental Illness.* London: Tavistock Publishers.

Wynne, L. and Singer, M. (1963). Thought disorder and family relations of schizophrenics (I and II). *Archives of General Psychiatry* 9:191-206.

Zigler, E. and Phillips, L. (1960). Social effectiveness and symptomatic behavior. *Journal of Abnormal and Social Psychology* 161: 231-238.

Zwerling, I. and Mendolsohn, M. (1965). Initial reactions to day hospitalization. *Family Process* 4(1): 50-63.

Chapter 7

Summary of Research Problems and Contributions of the Framework

This book undertook two related goals: to present a conceptual framework organizing clinical-service mental health research relevant to Hispanic populations in the United States and, in the context of this framework, to formulate a series of research problems. Before discussing the general features of the research problems and the contributions of the framework, three observations should be made.

The first pertains to the generalizability of the conceptual framework presented here. Although its development was prompted by the need for an integrated view of issues relevant to Hispanic mental health research, the framework is not linked uniquely either to mental health or to Hispanics. The minimal requirement for its use is the existence of institutions formally organized to solve or ameliorate the problems of individuals. Thus, the framework is equally applicable to health problems other than mental illness and to populations other than Hispanic. Questions can be asked about the rise of physical illness, how help is sought, how the illness is diagnosed and treated, and what experiences shape recovery after treatment. When asked sequentially, to coincide with the temporally arrayed phases, the questions serve as pointed reminders that the illness itself, whatever its character, has a history and that this history has been conditioned and shaped by the force of psychosocial and cultural factors.

The second observation is that the research problems are multidisciplinary in character. To formulate them, we have drawn from such diverse disciplines as sociology, anthropology, psychology, psychiatry, social work, and public health. Within these disciplines, different theoretical and methodological orientations have been considered in the conviction that problems of mental health—among Hispanics as well as other groups—are so multifaceted as to require the involvement of all the academic disciplines seeking to understand human behavior in its psychological and sociocultural context. We believe there is a need to depart radically from the compartmentalization of human knowledge which has resulted from the historical

139

demarcation of the boundaries of academic disciplines. The limits of mental health research questions and their corresponding rationales do not coincide with such discretely organized territories. Thus, there is a need to institutionalize an expanded multidisciplinary vision of mental health research.

The third observation calls attention to the need for programmatic research to address the research problems raised in this book. If there is a need for an expanded multidisciplinary vision, there is a need, too, to recognize that the complexities of mental health research do not yield to discrete research efforts. Each of the research problems warrants the attention of a series of research projects. How such projects should be integrated sequentially over time is itself problematical. But the problems cannot be resolved *a priori*, on the basis of some previously conceived overarching plan. The trajectories research follows are so often shaped by serendipitous findings as to defy long-range projections of what research should undertake. The issue of programmatic research clearly depends on the sensitivity of the research community to the accumulating legacies of research in defining promising avenues of inquiry. It is this sensitivity that we have attempted to employ in the formulation of research problems on Hispanic mental health.

The Research Problems

The first phase of the conceptual framework, focusing upon conditions associated with the rise of mental health problems, invites the formulation of broadly conceived epidemiological research which attempts to assess the distribution and severity of mental health problems among Hispanics in comparison to other groups. The common assumption that Hispanics disproportionately manifest mental health disorders still rests primarily upon inferences drawn from their demographic and experiential profile. Such inferences point to their generally low socioeconomic status, acculturative problems and, among first-generation Hispanics, the disruptions associated with the migration experience. The assumption is based, secondarily, upon the findings of studies which, using a variety of symptom lists, tend to show the existence of disproportionate psychological distress among Hispanics. Recognition has been given to the fact, however, that findings derived from such symptom lists do not, in and of themselves, yield clinical conclusions relevant to DSM III diagnostic categories.

Psychiatric epidemiology has sought to develop field-based techniques, such as the Diagnostic Interview Schedule, for the assessment of such diagnostic categories. The techniques still confront difficult psychometric problems, and their use with Hispanic populations has barely begun. One study conducted in Puerto Rico (Canino et al., 1987), however, indicated that the symptom-list findings showing the tendency for Puerto Ricans to experience disproportionate psychological distress are not congruent with findings based upon DSM III classifications, which show no such tendency. Conclusions on this issue are premature, but it is not premature to suggest that the absence of such congruity poses interesting questions relevant to Phase One. How do discrete symptoms, as reflected in symptom lists, become organized into diagnostic clinical configurations? Does the culture of Hispanic groups, and other ethnic groups, influence the first appearance of such symptoms and the subsequent processes leading to diagnostic configurations of these symptoms? These questions are substantive and point to the need for psychiatric epidemiology to engage more directly issues pertaining to the etiology of psychological distress.

In the pursuit of such objectives, we urge that the assessment of mental health be framed in terms of current symptoms and not from retrospective reports of lifetime mental health problems. The literature which has been cited and the discussion on mental health evaluation of Hispanics in Chapter 4 call attention to the numerous psychometric problems that arise when a subject's mental health is assessed at the time of the study. In epidemiological research even the temporal order of the administration of tests affects the findings derived from the tests; findings are affected, too, by the professional identity of the examiner or diagnostician. Mental health evaluations rely heavily upon the clients' self-reports of subjective states, implicating private feelings, perceptions, and experiences. Such reports must be viewed as expressions of the subjects' social constructions, which are endogenously shaped by culture, as clearly demonstrated by the research of Angel and Gronfein (1988). Thus, we confront the difficult measurement problem that equivalent scores on psychological tests may not have the same meaning for Hispanics as they do for non-Hispanics.

If such problems are evident in the evaluation of current mental health status, it follows that the problems associated with the assessment of lifetime prevalence rates are monumental, perhaps insurmountable. Such rates are so likely to be suffused with retrospectively based errors as to defy accurate interpretations. We recommend, therefore, that efforts to retrospectively assess lifetime mental health experiences surrender precedence to the implementation of prospectively organized longitudinal research capable of making accurate assessments of prevalence and incidence rates. The promise held by epidemiological research of providing reliable and valid data for the computation of such rates and solid clues as to the etiology of mental health distress remains largely unfulfilled in the study of Hispanic populations.

One step in the direction of fulfilling this promise is to orient epidemiological research toward the examination of migration-induced primary strains and the stress process, topics which correspond to the first phase's second and third research problems. The two topics can be dealt with by research either jointly or independently, since the stress process does not presuppose the migration experience. The stress process involves the relationship between life-event stresses and psychological distress, as mediated by social and intrapsychic resources in either migrant or non-migrant populations. However, when epidemiological research involves Hispanic groups with large proportions of first-generation immigrants—such as Puerto Ricans, Cubans, Dominicans, and Colombians—there is a distinct advantage in considering the topics jointly, as we did in Chapter 2: it provides an integrated and more comprehensive view of the processes intervening between migration-induced primary strains and psychological distress.

In developing such an integrated view, we have, first, eschewed the customary practice of listing in *ad hoc* fashion variables likely to be relevant to the connections between migration and mental health. Instead, we began the analysis by focusing upon the essential character of the migration experience: the changes resulting from being extracted from one socioeconomic system and inserted into another, the disruption of primary group bonds, and acculturative problems. Primary strains arise when the immigrant experiences downward social mobility into the bottom of the stratificational system and is subjected to the vicissitudes of economic cycles, when the primary bonds dissolved by the move to the new sociocultural system are slow to be restored, when the immigrant is either acculturatively isolated or projected precipitously into the host society, away from a functional bicultural modality. It is imperative that research keep primary strains analytically distinct from the stresses induced by life-event changes, which represent one component in the usual formulations of the stress process. In contrast to life-event changes which occur in a circumscribed period of time and tend to be episodic, migration-induced primary strains deeply envelop large segments of the immigrant's life for prolonged periods of time. The concept of primary strain represents an attempt to capture changes organically rooted in the migration experience which are likely to have broad and deleterious effects upon the Hispanic immigrant's psychological well-being. The concept is obviously applicable to other immigrant groups as well.

Primary strains impinge separately or jointly, directly or indirectly, upon the immigrant's mental health. This proposition embodies a complex set of interlocking, temporally ordered hypotheses which can be deduced from the figure presented in Chapter 2. The hypotheses call attention to the possible individual and interactive effects of primary strains upon components of the stress process, and the possibility of such effects in linkages between such components and psychological distress. For example, what is the character of life-event changes experienced by first-generation Hispanic immigrants located at the bottom of the stratification heap, shorn of their intimate and traditional family bonds, and experiencing the acculturative problems of linguistic isolation from the broader institutions of the host society? Under such circumstances, do life-event changes become more compressed, volatile, and unmanageable? We believe that the effect of such primary strains upon life events is likely to be more than additive, in fact, interactive, and that the impact which the events have upon psychological distress is profoundly deleterious. Questions such as this, and others too, derive from the formulations which have been presented. The questions can be raised but they cannot be answered here. Once again, there is a need for prospectively-oriented epidemiological studies which begin with primary strains and extend forward into the life cycle of immigrant groups.

Phase Two examines the help-seeking efforts prompted by the emergence of mental health problems. In the formulation of the two research problems in this phase, we focused our questions upon Hispanics who have contacted official mental health providers, as well as those not having such contacts but needing them. The concept of underutilization of mental health facilities, which is at the core of the first research problem, has been defined and measured in a variety of ways. But one of the most important defining elements has been largely neglected: information about the need for mental health services as reflected in true rates of mental health problems. The assertion that Hispanics underutilize services, although very plausible, must still be treated as a promising hypothesis in need of systematic testing.

This hypothesis, which is at the core of the first research problem, becomes part of the broader theoretical structure implicated by the second research problem which outlines the major explanations for Hispanics' purported underutilization of mental health facilities. The first explanation is that Hispanics cope with or contain their mental health problems within their own primary indigenous organizations, as an alternative to official care; and the second is that they experience barriers to mental health care which are located within Hispanic culture or in the institutional characteristics of the mental health care delivery system. Research has touched upon aspects of both explanations, but now it is possible to delineate in a much more comprehensive way than before the requirements of research: data on the true prevalence or incidence of mental health distress, measures reflecting the degree of integration into alternative indigenous organizations, measures of acculturation, assessments of the institutional features of the available mental health facilities, and utilization rates. The structure of the second research problem is clear if we take the last component to signify the criterion variable to be explained, and theoretically order the first four components—a procedure which is quite plausible—to test for their independent or interactive effects on utilization. The inferential power of such research is enhanced substantially, once again, if the research is prospectively organized and longitudinal in character, since the problem being addressed is a process, namely, help-seeking. In such an effort, there is a distinct role to be played by qualitatively oriented research to develop hypotheses relevant to the specific interconnections between components.

From a research viewpoint, the classification or measurement of mental health problems commences at the very beginning of the first phase, as we have seen in our discussion of psychiatric epidemiology, and retains research relevance throughout the phases of the framework. However, from the viewpoint of psychologically distressed Hispanics traversing the phases, the assessment of mental health attains institutional significance in the third phase after the initial contacts have been made with mental health officials. In this setting, the vast diagnostic technologies of the clinical and social sciences are brought to bear upon the distressed client with the resulting imposition of diagnostic labels. Very likely, the client has brought into this setting his or her own labels, representing attempts to understand the distress, as a by-product of previous help-seeking interactions in indigenous, primary social groups. But it is the imprint of the official or professionally sanctified label which now attains extraordinary significance in shaping the client's future life trajectory. How accurate are such labels in capturing the Hispanics' experience of psychological distress? How adequately and extensively do the labels comprehend Hispanics' problems of distress? Most importantly, are the assumptions underlying the assignment of clinical labels congruous with their culture and life situation? In the client's life, answers to these questions are consequential.

The two research problems imbedded in the third phase represent efforts to answer these questions, each invoking troublesome issues in the mental health assessment of Hispanics. The first focuses upon the attributes, procedures, and assumptions of the long-standing, widely used psychological tests administered to Hispanics. The testing literature has identified multiple sources of test bias, ranging from those which implicate the failure to develop culturally appropriate performance norms to those stemming from the non-equivalence of measures across ethnic groups, issues to which we previously alluded. The failure to test Hispanics adequately is distressing, considering the unmet prescriptions of psychological testing standards. The research problem documents the pressing need to bring the testing of Hispanics to conform to such standards.

While the first research problem in Phase Three focuses upon instrumentation biases, the second considers biases resulting from situational factors impinging upon the evaluation of mental health. To appreciate the real-life background of the problem it is helpful to imagine the vast number of situations which bring together distressed Hispanics and diagnosticians in mental health facilities across the United States. In all of these situations, diagnosis is reached by taking into consideration much more than the clients' psychological condition. According to current research findings, other factors impinge upon the diagnosis: the language spoken (Spanish or English) during the diagnostic interview, the client's language dominance (Spanish or English), and the ethnicity of the diagnostician (Hispanic or non-Hispanic). Each factor is suffused with cultural meaning and, when considered together, they reflect the generalized cultural distance or proximity between client and diagnostician. The second research problem poses questions about the interrelationship of such factors in shaping the client's communication of symptoms and the diagnostician's interpretation of such communications in the evaluation of mental health. The problem's institutional importance is matched by the inconclusiveness of current research findings. It invites the attention of studies oriented toward situations in which diagnoses are made, as well as experimentally oriented laboratory research.

In Phase Four diagnosis has been completed and therapy has begun and will continue until the client withdraws from treatment, often by just failing to keep appointments, or when judgments are made either by the client, the therapist or both that the therapeutic improvements can no longer be expected. Premature withdrawal from treatment, often referred to as the problem of attrition, is commonplace among Hispanic clients. But even if the client remains in treatment, there is no assurance that the treatment is sensitive to the client's culture. In fact, the pervasive practice and policy has been to bring traditional therapeutic modalities, developed in middle-class populations, to bear upon the emotional problems of members of minority ethnic groups with little or no alteration in the format of delivery. This, in fact, is the crux of the generally accepted isomorphic assumption that therapy should mirror the client's culture, out of which the two research problems in Phase Four were formulated. The plea for cultural sensitivity in the administration of treatment should also be a plea for the development of research focusing upon the effectiveness of culturally sensitized treatments.

The research problems grew out of an examination of clinical reports dealing with Hispanics and our own analysis of what it means to say that treatments have been rendered culturally sensitive. As the first research problem implies, the usual meaning calls for the selection and modification of therapies strictly according to the client's culture. This procedure is straightforward and direct, and is most clearly and comprehensively exemplified in the research on Cubans discussed in Chapter 5. The mandate is for cultural isomorphism: Cubans are familiocentric; therefore, the therapist selects family therapy. Cubans are strongly oriented toward hierarchical interpersonal structures; therefore, the therapy is modified to situate the therapist in a position of authority. Compliance with the mandate sets the stage for dealing with the isomorphic issue, not as an axiom, but as a hypothesis well worth the attention given to it by the first research problem of Phase Four. The research question becomes: Are therapies selected and modified to mirror the client's culture more therapeutically effective than those which are neither selected nor modified on cultural grounds?

The second research problem departs from the isomorphic assumption and opens up the way for a broader vision of what cultural sensitivity entails. It considers the hypothesis that therapeutic gains can sometimes be made when traditional cultural patterns are bent, changed, or redirected according to the therapeutic goals. The hypothesis assumes that the client's culture can be respected without being isomorphically replicated in therapy. One study, cited in Chapter 5, provides compelling experimental evidence in support of such departures. In order to modify a treatment program according to the needs of a cultural group, research hypotheses must be carefully developed to reflect the intricacies of the many possible connections between various cultural traits and the therapies being administered. Research seeking to test such hypotheses may well indicate the value of sometimes preserving, sometimes counteracting, and sometimes altering the client's adherence to traditional cultural elements. The ultimate aim should be the adaptation of the Hispanic client to the host society in such a way that ethnic identity and pride are not negated or belied.

The first chapter called attention to macro societal changes impinging upon Hispanics who are experiencing the processes delineated by the framework's five phases. Changes in mental health policy and in the family structure of some Hispanic groups create the research problems in Phase Five. For example, the sweeping effect of the deinstitutionalization movement coincides historically with the increasing number of single-parent house-holds among Puerto Rican and Dominican families. The families are in-creasingly unable to assume the supportive functions relevant to aftercare. Thus, the changes have added complexity to the post-treatment phase and, at the same time, broadened the range of relevant research questions.

The two research problems in this phase represent a set of questions about the post-treatment experience of Hispanics suffering from a serious mental illness. Some of the questions seek descriptive information: How many are rehospitalized? How many return to their families or are placed in other settings? How many are homeless? Do Hispanics contact agencies and seek mental health or vocational rehabilitation? The number of descriptive ques-tions could be multiplied over and over. So could the questions about His-panics' reintegration into the family and the community, and their involve-ment in aftercare mental health programs. But the information to answer both types of questions is so conspicuously absent as to prevent the formula-tion of more subtly constructed research problems. The need is clear: large-scale descriptively or analytically oriented research seeking to trace the af-tercare experience of Hispanics and other ethnic groups.

At the risk of repeating previous recommendations, it is important to em-phasize the need for cultural sensitivity in conducting the research proposed in the five phases. This need, in fact, remains largely unfulfilled in studies examining the life circumstances giving rise to emotional distress; how such distress prompts help-seeking efforts; the convergence of sociocultural forces upon the evaluation of mental health status; the intricate adaptations of therapies to clients; and the effectiveness of such therapies in enabling the rehabilitation of clients. Cultural sensitivity is not a matter of an occa-sional adaptation or insertion into the research process. It is needed in the planning and pretesting of research, in the collection of data and translation of instruments, in the instrumentation of measures, and in the analysis and interpretation of data. This means that there should be an incessant and continuing finely calibrated interweaving of cultural components and cul-tural awareness in all phases of the research process (Rogler, 1989).

We have seen that the framework temporally orders research. What other contributions does it make?

Contributions of the Conceptual Framework

The hypothetical temporal sequence with its unfolding five-phase struc-ture is the framework's organizing principle. This serves as a persistent re-minder that human experiences associated with the emergence of emotional problems (or other maladies) and efforts to cope with such problems, whether personal or institutional, inevitably occur in the context of time-driven social processes. But few, indeed, are the mental health studies which depart from simple cross-sectional assessments. Typically but implicitly, the research proceeds as if such experiences were frozen in time, suspended in history, with no past or future. The multiplication of cross-sectional mental health studies, progressively accumulating larger sets of ahistorical find-ings, will continue to constrict and confuse our understanding of processes relevant to mental health. Efforts aimed at the prevention of psychological disorders also will be deleteriously affected. After all, the various forms of prevention are rooted in the very same temporal process we have attempted to define: primary, seeking to decrease the occurrence of new cases of psy-chological disorder; secondary, seeking to attenuate or cure the disorder; and tertiary, attempting to reduce the disabling impact of the disorder and its harmful consequences through rehabilitation. The framework's temporal sequence and the individualized attention we have given to the phases' re-search problems represent attempts to give explicit meaning and emphasis to the customary plea for longitudinally oriented studies.

The distinctions between phases in the framework accentuate the need to make corresponding distinctions in the formulation of some research problems. Thus, in the epidemiological studies cited in Phase One, rates of treated prevalence often were used as a proxy for rates of true prevalence. Our discussion of Phases One and Two shows that to confound such statis-tics easily leads to errors in research and possible misjudgment in mental health policy. The Phase Two research problems indicated that statistics based upon the records of treatment facilities represent the outcome of com-plicated community-based processes. More than likely, such treatment sta-tistics do not have a stable correlation with true prevalence or incidence rates across demographic, social, and cultural groups in the population at large (Vernon and Roberts, 1982). The implications of this issue are likely to be more deleterious in the formulation of mental health policy for minori-ty groups to the extent that such groups tend to be underutilizers. For this reason, the analytical distinction between Phases One and Two should be kept in mind: the first ends with the existence of a psychological problem, the second begins with it.

Nonetheless, findings from one phase can contribute to solving the re-search problems in subsequent phases. To return to the previous point as an example, in the transition of research from Phase One to Phase Two, true prevalence or incidence rates are essential to evaluating the frequency of ethnic group utilization of mental health facilities. Thus, we avoid simplistic conclusions about over- or underutilization among ethnic groups (such as Hispanics) based only on comparisons between the proportion of users of mental health facilities who belong to a specific ethnic group and the proportionate size of that ethnic group in the facilities' catchment area. As the discussion of Phase Two indicated, such comparisons do not take into account the need factor, as exemplified by true prevalence, in the delivery of mental health care. Other examples could be provided of how findings in one phase can be projected usefully toward the examination of problems in subsequent phases. For instance, the assessment of mental health, Phase Three, is directly relevant to the specification of "outcome" measures in the evaluation of Phase Four treatment modalities. The sequential ordering of the phases signifies that each phase contains antecedent variables relevant to the research problems in successive phases.

If the relevance of variables often is transferable from one phase to a subsequent one, so are some of the explanatory schemes developed for research problems in different phases. Thus in Phase Two research problems, explanations for variations in the utilization of mental health facilities by Hispanics were premised upon alternative resource and barrier theories. As we have seen, the former theory posits the relevance of primary group networks in ameliorating or containing the mental health problems of its members, whereas the latter theory points to cultural and institutional impediments to the use of mental health facilities. The root problem is to explain how persons get attached or fail to get attached to institutional structures delivering mental health care. The same problem appears in Phase Five, in considering how seriously mentally ill Hispanics can be induced to make use of aftercare mental health programs. The problem being the same, the same theories are brought to bear upon it, with the exception that the Phase Five client now has had a life history experience of having traversed through the phases.

Earlier in this chapter we mentioned the importance of accurate mental health assessments, an issue discussed in Chapter 4. Without culturally appropriate measurement scales of psychiatric symptoms or psychodiagnostic procedures attuned to the patients' language and culture, epidemiological studies of true or treated prevalence rates cannot provide an accurate assessment of mental illness patterns in Hispanic populations. Without accurate assessment and diagnosis, and without the knowledge of whether psychological evaluations are distorted in the direction of over- or underestimation of illness, we lose our grasp of the mental health needs of Hispanics, which is one of the goals of Phase One research. Similarly, allegations of underutilization of services by Hispanics, in the Phase Two literature, are premised on accurate estimates of prevalence rates or mental health needs. Subsequent to Phase Three, the diagnosis rendered is presumed to shape the course of psychotherapeutic intervention. Treatments in Phase Four will be misdirected to the extent that they reflect inappropriate perceptions of the nature and severity of the patient's disorder. These reverberations of Phase Three issues are evident in Phase Five, as mental health problems re-emerge, as services are once again sought, and as the assessment and treatment processes are re-administered. The problem of evaluating the rehabilitation of discharged patients is magnified if the original evaluation of the patient is dubious. The use of the framework serves as a persistent reminder that the accurate assessment of psychological distress is an issue whose importance transcends all phases of epidemiological and clinical services research.

There are other contributions the framework makes, some of which have been alluded to, others not. As seen in our discussion of the fifth phase, it identifies major gaps in research. No argument should be made calling for an equal distribution of research efforts across the five phases. However, the persistent neglect of issues pertinent to the post-treatment rehabilitation of Hispanic clients, in the context of the deinstitutionalization movement and the rise of community mental health clinics in previously unserved inner-city neighborhoods, has denied us a research base for the formulation of intelligent public policy and practice focusing upon rehabilitation. The framework's capacity to detect such neglect stems from its easy conversion into a practical scheme for classifying bibliographical items. In the language of content analysis, each of the five phases can be treated as a content category and the specific bibliographical item as a content unit classified into the appropriate category (Berelson, 1952). We applied this procedure to bibliographies of Hispanic mental health research and were able to detect the lacunae of research in Phase Five.

The first chapter briefly foreshadowed the importance of cultural concepts in understanding the clinical experiences of Hispanic clients. What was foreshadowed there was amplified in subsequent chapters. Thus, acculturation was postulated to be a critical mediator between migration and the emergence of mental health distress. It was also seen to play a role in shaping the help-seeking effort prompted by such distress, and in forming contacts with mental health facilities. In the evaluation of mental health, the concept of acculturation was inserted into the effort to resolve psychometric problems of mental health instruments and scales pervasively biased toward majority middle-class white populations, and it was seen to shed light on clinical situations distorting the mental health evaluation of Hispanics. Problems associated with the selection, modification, and development of mental health treatment modalities with Hispanics were framed according to the isomorphic assumption that there ought to be a mirrorlike relationship between therapy and the client's culture; experimental evidence was shown to support the need for testing hypotheses departing from the assumption by taking into account the intermingling between the client's traditional culture and the culture of the host society. And, although the literature on Phase Five is scarce, acculturative elements appear to play an important role in the rehabilitation of Hispanic clients. In brief, the framework enables the identification over time of the likely continuing influence of acculturation. In turn, the importance of acculturation transcends the five phases because it signifies experiences fundamentally rooted in the Hispanics' integration into the host society's culture.

However, we are in agreement with Marsella and Takeuchi's statement (1987) that most mental health professionals remain oblivious to the importance of culture in the planning and development of mental health services for minority populations. Nor is the "potency" of this concept understood, as they also state. In the interest of addressing the problem of ignorance and the need to enhance our understanding, we propose that the acculturative process itself be the object of basic research: it should be commonly recognized that any scientific increment in our knowledge of the acculturative process represents a corresponding increment in our understanding of the mental health of Hispanics and other immigrant minority groups. Toward this end, we make three broad research proposals.

First, research should conceive of acculturation as two processes which can be analytically distinguished but which are empirically interrelated: involvements in the traditional culture and involvements in the host society culture. Psychometrically appropriate measures of acculturation should explicitly reflect this distinction in the interest of examining how these dual processes interrelate. In developing hypotheses as to how they interrelate, simplistic assumptions of a linear progression away from traditional culture and toward host society culture ought to be avoided. It is not likely that the acquisition of one cultural element is followed by the corresponding loss of the element in the other culture. A functional admixture of both cultures, in fact, is likely to be a frequent modality and one which is less stressful than precipitous departures from traditional culture and precipitous insertions into host society culture. This formulation undergirds the bicultural hypothesis advanced in Phase One and makes the hypothesis more plausible than others which postulate a simple direct or inverse relationship between acculturation and mental health problems.

The second proposal is that research should conceive of such processes as containing multiple factors or diverse cultural elements. Language is involved, and so are values, preferences, habits, customs, and self-concept. By recognizing the multifaceted character of the processes, we can see that change across the elements is not likely to be uniform, that it will likely favor some elements over others. Acculturative change proceeds unevenly. When research focuses upon how the change occurs, some theoretical assumptions can be brought into the effort. Thus, in a study of intergenerational processes in Puerto Rican families living in New York City, Rogler and Cooney (1984) used the concepts of instrumental and expressive elements to theorize about such change. The learning of the host society's language, for example, is instrumental because it is avowedly goal-directed. On the other hand, the persons' subjective ethnic identity, as part of the self-concept, is an expressive element because it is a private, psychological by-product of social experiences. The theory is that instrumental elements, being located more at the interface of cross-cultural contacts than expressive elements, will change more rapidly than the expressive elements. The theory fits the intergenerational acculturative changes of the Puerto Rican families. Even though the theory is rudimentary, it is sufficiently promising to invite the attention of future research.

The third proposal is that research be mindful of the fact that acculturation occurs and unfolds in a socioeconomic and cultural context. The socioeconomic context is important because socioeconomic status is directly related to acculturation (Rogler and Cooney, 1984) and, as seen in Phase One, it is inversely related to the prevalence of mental health problems. Research examining the relationship between acculturation and mental illness should first account for the influence of socioeconomic status and consider the distinct possibility that the dynamics of acculturative change previously mentioned may be conditioned by socioeconomic status. Assessments of the cultural environment—the plurality of ethnic groups in the setting, their size, and institutional dominance—should also form part of the research. It is this environment which gives meaning to the direction of acculturative change. Research findings (Rogler and Cooney, 1984) suggest that when familally linked generations share the same culture in their early socialization, there tends to be more intergenerational continuity in acculturation. The complexity of these ideas should be matched by the complexity of the research effort which addresses them. The effort is needed because acculturation emerges as a concept of paramount importance in understanding the mental health experience of Hispanics as they traverse the five phases of the framework.

We have seen that the conceptual framework is generalizable to other forms of illness and other ethnic groups, temporally orders research problems, accentuates important research distinctions which coincide with changes from one phase to the next, illustrates the transferable relevance of variables and of explanatory schemes from one phase to the next, serves as a reminder that the accurate measurement of psychological distress is a problem in all phases of clinical research, identifies gaps in research, and situates important concepts within the mental health experience of Hispanics. It can make another contribution too: in a metaphorical sense the temporally arrayed phases serve as successive filters from the first to the last phase. Among Hispanics confronting the risks described in Phase One, how many succumb to problems of mental health? Among those with such problems, how many go through the help-seeking processes delineated in Phase Two and terminate with contacts with mental health facilities? Among those who form such contacts, how many have their mental health problem validly diagnosed in Phase Three? Among these with such diagnosis, how many receive appropriate mental health treatment in Phase Four? Among those who have received such treatment, how many in Phase Five experience reintegration into the community and utilize aftercare services? If we had research-based knowledge pertinent to the entire filtration process, and the associated ramifications, we would then have a holistic appreciation of what it is like, as a minority person with a different language and culture, to successively confront the grim realities underlying the metaphor.

References

Angel, R. and Gronfein, W. (1988). The use of subjective information in statistical models. *American Sociological Review* 53: 464-473.

Berelson, B. (1952). *Content Analysis in Communication Research.* Glencoe, Ill.: The Free Press.

Canino, G.J., Bird, H.R., Shrout, P.E., Rubio-Stipec, M., Bravo, M., Martinez, R. Sesman, M., and Guevara, L.M. (1987). The prevalence of specific psychiatric disorders in Puerto Rico. *Archives of General Psychiatry* 727-735.

Marsella, A.J. and Takeuchi, D.T. (August 1987). Reaction paper: Pacific Islander perspective. *Minority Mental Health Services Research Conference Proceedings.* Minority Research Resources Branch, Division of Biometry and Applied Sciences, National Institute of Mental Health.

Rogler, L.H. (1989). The meaning of culturally sensitive research in mental health. *American Journal of Psychiatry* 146(4).

Rogler, L.H. and Cooney, R.S. (1984). *Puerto Rican Families in New York City: Intergenerational Processes.* Maplewood, N.J.: Waterfront Press (Hispanic Research Center Monograph No. 11).

Vernon, S.W. and Roberts, R.E. (1982). Prevalence of treated psychiatric disorders in three ethnic groups. *Social Science Medicine* 16: 1575-1582.

Subject Index

Author Index

Abad, V. 54,56,59,65
Acosta, F. 100,114
Adebimpe, V.R. 84,90
Alers, J.O. 48,65
Ames, L.M. 81,91
Amin, A.E. 127,132
Anastasi, A. 81,91
Anderson, C.M. 125,127,132
Anderson, G. 81,91
Anderson, H. 81,91
Aneshensel, C. 25,37,78,91
Angel, R. 36,38,141,153
Anthony, W.A. 129,132
Arce, C.J. 27,41
Arenas, S. 54,65
Argulewicz, E.N. 80,91
Atwood, N. 125,132
August, J. 81,91

Bachrach, S. 47,65
Baekland, F. 100,115
Bailey, B.E. 82,91
Barrera, M. 62,65
Barrow, S. 130,132
Baskin, D. 17,38
Bateson, G. 126,132
Bean, L.L. 124,125,135
Beels, C.C. 125,132
Beiser, M. 130,132
Bell, R.A. 25,38

Berelson, B. 150,153
Berry, J.W. 33,38
Bessuk, E.L. 120,132
Bettelheim, B. 112,115
Billings, A.G. 25,38
Birley, J.L. 33,38,125,132
Bloom, B. 61,65
Bluestone, H. 54,56,65,104,115
Booth, L.J. 81,91
Boulette, T.R. 110,115
Boureston, N.C. 126,133
Bozlee, S. 76,95
Brameld, T. 51,66
Bromet, E. 25,38
Brown, G. 33,38,125,126,132,133
Burnam, M.A. 27,38
Butcher, J.H. 77,91

Canino, G.J. 18,19,38,39,141,153
Carkhuff, R. 85,91
Carpenter, J.D. 126,133
Carpenter, W.T. 125,136
Casas, J.M. 54,59,62,68
Casas, M.E. 103,116
Castro, F.G. 29,30,33,34,35,39,54, 56,66
Catalano, R. 4,10,23,24,39
Cervantes, R.C. 29,30,33,34,35,39
Chesney, A.P. 57,66
Clark, L.A. 77,91